HEALTH CARE FOR PLUS FIFTY

Dr O.P. Jaggi, a renowned physician and a medical scientist of international standing, is a crusader in the field of demystifying medicine and medical facts for the benefit of the common man. He firmly believes in the concept of preventive medicine and, therefore, in explaining medical facts. He has published a multi-volume encyclopaedia of medicine, and his over a dozen books on health-care are immensely popular. During his professional life extending over 30 years, he has travelled widely and studied health problems under different environments. He has been Senior Consultant Physician to the Govt. of Nigeria; Dean of Faculty of Medical Sciences, University of Delhi; and Director, V. Patel Chest Institute, Delhi. He is President of the Foundation of Total Health Care.

HEALTH CARE
FOR
PLUS FIFTY

Dr. O.P. Jaggi, M.D., Ph.D.
F.C.C.P. (USA), F.A.C.A. (USA)
F.R.A.S. (London)

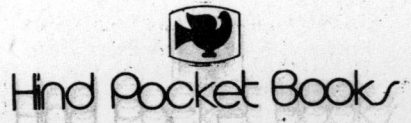

Hind Pocket Books

HEALTH CARE FOR PLUS FIFTY
© Dr. O.P. Jaggi, 1991
First paperback edition, 1991
This paperback edition, 1998
ISBN 81-216-0203-3

Published by
Hind Pocket Books (P) Ltd.
18-19, Dilshad Garden, G.T. Road
Delhi-110 095

Designing, Typesetting
& Print Production : SCANSET
18-19, Dilshad Garden, G.T., Road, Delhi-110 095
Tel: 228 2467, 229 7792, 93, 94   Fax: 228 2332

Printed at Nice Printing Press, Delhi-110 051

PRINTED IN INDIA

Preface

From time immemorial, people have sung praises to the wonder of youth and bemoaned the woes of old age. Youth is equated with health and old age with disease.

Old age has also been equated with wisdom, experience and respect of the society.

Taking the above two facets together, it seems, if we can prevent or curb disease in old age, this period of life can be more satisfying and more worth living.

This brings us to the question: what brings on ageing? Many theories have been propounded in this regard. I would, however, like to quote a relevant passage from *Charaka Samhita*, an ancient Ayurvedic text. It states:

> All ills of the body arise...in consumers of sour, salt, pungent and alkaline articles, dried vegetables, flesh...softened, heavy, stale foods, meals taken at irregular times or in irregular quantities or too frequently, i.e., over a stomach that has not yet recovered from the last meal, addicts to day-sleeping, sex pleasures and wine bibbing, persons whose bodies have been strained by faulty or inordinate indulgence in exercise; and victims of fear, anger, grief, greed, infatuation and overwork....
>
> Therefore, having regard to such ills, one should give up the above-mentioned unwholesome diet and regimen.

Charaka's above remarks have been substantiated by the latest findings of modern medicine.

In spite of all the precautions, old age is still susceptible to many diseases, some of which are due to the normal wear and tear of the body. While these diseases may not be easily cured, yet they can be managed.

This book divided into three parts describes the process of ageing, managing old age in general, and recognition and treatment of specific diseases.

My qualifications for writing such a book are: a medical career extending over four decades and my age which is plus sixty. I hope the readers will find the book useful.

—O.P. Jaggi

Contents

Introduction

Ageing was certainly a fun for one of our neighbours, Mr. Gopal Das. He was seventy-one years young. I call him young because there wasn't anything old about him except a good crop of snow-white hair on his head, which he kept covered with his white turban. He wore his turban inside his house, too, even while he was not wearing shoes. He was president of the area Welfare Committee and I remember, during the Pakistani conflict in 1965, he had kept vigil of the area for four nights along with his sons, grandsons, and others. He liked everybody and everybody liked him. To meet people and gossip with them was his hobby, and being a property-dealer, he combined business with pleasure. He enjoyed life. He liked good food and almost all his life he had overeaten. He had diabetes and once a minor brain stroke also. On the insistence of his relatives, he went to a doctor who advised him to reduce his weight by cutting down his diet. Mr. Gopal Das did not like the doctor nor his advice and so never went to another again.

Personally I think he should have followed the advice of this doctor, and I will tell you why.

Diet

Recently, a nutrition expert carried out an interesting experiment in his laboratory. He divided 300 newly weaned rats into three groups. To group A rats, he gave a less than average but an otherwise well-balanced diet. To group B, he fed a very rich diet giving them as much as they could take. Group C rats were given a diet similar to that of B group, but they were confined in specially built cages, so that there was very little opportunity for them to move about much.

The results were startling. While group A rats fed on less than the average diet lived for more than 1500 days, group B rats who had rich diet lived for about a thousand days, and the rats in group C who also had heavy diet but with restricted movement survived only for 750 days.

These and similar experiments have proved conclusively that the nutritional pattern and mode of living are important factors that control the life of an individual, even more than the heredity does.

Over-eating and consequent increase in weight is one of the factors that leads to development of heart attacks, high blood pressure, brain strokes, diabetes, and diseases of the kidneys. Ill-health in later years due to these and many other diseases is not merely the result of growing old, but, among other factors, is due to the long-drawn dietary indiscretions of youth and middle age. Statistics gathered from Insurance Companies show that between the ages of forty and forty-five, over-weight begins to tell upon health. An excess of 12.5 kg. for instance lessens the expectation of life by 25 per cent and a further increase is even worse.

It is important to remember that this is entirely preventable, and for this, the first thing to do is to avoid overeating. What is important is not the amount of food eaten, but a well-balanced diet. Lean and wiry individuals are known to eat less but they keep physically fit till a very old age. While over-weight people who reduce to the normal weight for their age, can have an almost normal life expectancy, it is easier to avoid putting on weight than to reduce it later. I am reminded of a nutrition expert who helped his patients reduce their weight by a technique he had learnt by experience. On enquiry, his patients would invariably tell him of the little food they took, in spite of which they were increasing in weight. He would note down carefully the diet which the patient said he/she usually took. Then he would call the nurse-in-charge and instruct her to admit the patient in the ward and put him or her on the same diet as mentioned by the patient. All his patients lost upto 5 kgs. of weight in three weeks on that diet! This proves clearly that one can overeat without being aware of doing so.

Physical Exercise

The role of daily physical exercise in maintaining good health is equally important. Like the rats in group C of the experiment, people who do little physical exercise, await the same fate. In our sedentary civilization, a person generally confined to a chair in the office possesses a heart in his thirties which should normally belong to one in his fifties. From our point of view, the significant observation is that regular exercise can restore such hearts to a near-normal condition.

Mental Health

While physical health is necessary to enjoy the growing years, this in itself is not enough. One needs to remain active and mentally alert as well. There is no truth in the statement that mental powers normally decline as one grows older. Such an impression in the past was created by comparing the mental performance of twenty-year olds with those in the fifty-year group. This naturally gave inaccurate results because twenty-year olds were more educated and informed because of the better facilities available to them than were available to those in their fifties when they were young. More recent follow-up studies of the same individual at the ages twenty and fifty-five have shown that mental alertness and receptivity generally increases with age. Mental sluggishness, on the other hand, is the outcome of the continual rusting of unused faculties.

Examples of elderly people who take courses of study and do extremely well are seen increasingly at university convocations. Such people are really too busy to let their minds grow old. They defy the ravages of time and stay young despite the wrinkles on their faces.

Multiple Interests

Old age is no bar to enjoying and finding satisfaction in life and also in being a useful citizen. But for this, one must cultivate interest in activities which give pleasure and satisfaction. A person need not follow only one profession or a way of life throughout his life. A teacher need not remain a teacher always, a doctor remain a doctor always, and a businessman or a shopkeeper remain in his restricted environment always. A doctor who is a bit of an artist, or a businessman with an interest in scientific subjects, would be a greater asset to society. With some people two or more interests or professions go very well indeed. Such interests are challenging and, taken up in moderation, go a long way in keeping one mentally active, so that when one retires one does not feel lost, but, in fact, is relieved and can pursue other activities.

For Old Grand-parents

Now a few words about those who are in the still older age group, the grand-parents. Experience has shown that if they keep themselves busy with some regular work, they find life more satisfying and thus they are a source of comfort and joy to others as well. I know an old man in our village who had been a farmer. But now he was not equal to the hard exertion of farming and his sons had taken over. The old man could not sit idle. In his youth, he had learnt the job of a carpenter. Now he would go to people's houses in the village and mend their *charpoys* free. If, on some day nobody needed his help, he would sit under a tree and make little playthings and distribute them among the children. They loved to collect around him and request him to make something for them.

My own grandfather used to keep a little shop, but in later years he retired from his work. In his early life, he had learnt to make a special kind of ointment for boils, which was known to be very useful in the days when the modern miracle drugs were not known. I remember him smearing the ointment on a small piece of round white cloth and applying it to the boils of the young and the old. He would do this in the mornings and rest in the evenings. His total expenditure per month was only five rupees. But this petty sum and the time and labour well spent, gave him great satisfaction right upto old age.

People with different interests can do the same. A retired teacher, a lawyer, or a doctor and others can help people around them by rousing or maintaining their interest in various matters and thus promote their zest for living. It is unhealthy for an old man to curb his interests and be a bore to himself and others. He should still have widening interests just like a river which starts as a rivulet and grows larger and wider as it goes ahead towards the sea.

The Process of Ageing

1 Changes in the Body due to Ageing

As one grows older, changes occur in the body. These changes may be categorised as:

(1) External, i.e., those which are visible,

(2) Internal, i.e., those which occur in the internal organs of the body, and

(3) Sense organ perceptions.

It is very important to know and recognize the changes that occur normally with ageing, because this knowledge helps one to distinguish a particular symptom, sign or result of a test in an older person as normal due to ageing, or abnormal due to a disease. Furthermore, it helps in proper understanding of the behaviour and response of an aged person.

External Changes

These are seen most obviously in the hair, face, skin, stature and posture, bony joints, mobility, etc.

Hair

One of the most obvious features of an older person is the greying of the hair. The hair also tends to become sparse. Baldness, of course, is common in men, but even in women there may be a considerable thinning of the hair.

Face

The muscles of expression and emotion are responsible for the characteristic wrinkling produced in time. Habitual patterns of expression, such as frowning, pursing the mouth, and smiling, produce characteristic wrinkles in some persons earlier in life than in others. Their onset is determined by factors such as toughness and elasticity of the skin, exposure to solar radiation, the extent

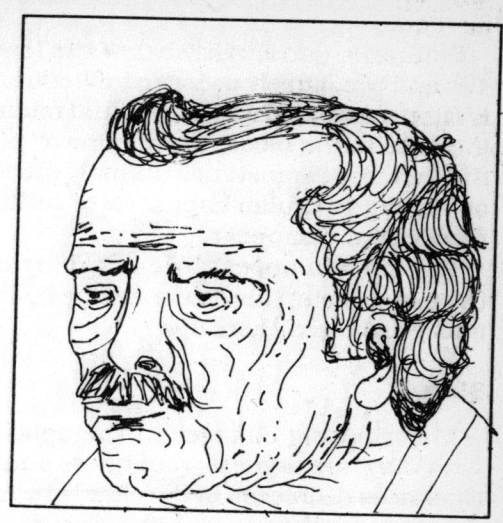

Wrinkles of old age

to which subcutaneous fat is maintained during ageing, and the state of nutrition.

Among the first wrinkles to form are those on the forehead. They start in the 20s and increase in the 30s and 40s; the initially thin tracings become deeper and thicker with the passage of years. Alongwith them develop wrinkles that radiate fan-wise from the lateral angle of the eye, known as crow's feet. Other facial wrinkles include those involving the angles of the mouth and the lips.

In addition to the progressive wrinkling, creasing results from the loss of fat and elastic fibres in the ageing skin. This leads to a laxness of skin, which then drapes itself chiefly in accordance with gravitational pull and produces a hanging down (ptosis) of lids, ears, jowls. In a few persons, sagging of the tissues of the neck combined with fat deposition produces a double chin. More often the neck undergoes shrinking and wrinkling, that may become even more marked than the facial changes.

Besides the wrinkles and the creases, there are other changes in the face as well. Loss of teeth progressively, leads to resorption of bone from the mandible and maxilla. When advanced, this produces marked shrinkage in the lower portion of the face, an increased infolding of the mouth, and shortened distance between the chin and nose. A slight elongation of the nose has also been recorded.

In many elderly persons, the skin of the face appears pale with little or no evidence of reddish tinge over such areas as the cheeks, and indeed the bloodless tone might at first glance suggest anaemia.

Puffiness, particularly below the lower lids, may develop in the 40s and 50s, largely owing to infilteration of fat into the area, which is often associated with some fluid retention. When associated with increase in the blood in the veins or pigmentation, this produces the dark bags sometimes unjustly attributed to keeping late hours or having irregular habits; later in life these, however, seem to recede and disappear.

The sunken appearance of elderly eyes is due to loss of fat in the eye sockets; this can be severe by the time the 70s are reached and progresses thereafter.

Skin

Major ageing changes in the appearance of the skin, besides wrinkling, are dryness, roughness and uneven pigmentation. Skin thickness decreases in the elderly by as much as 20 per cent. This accounts for the paper-thin, sometimes nearly transparent quality of their skin. The age-associated loss of blood vessels is believed to underlie many of the physiologic alterations in old skin, as well as the gradual atrophy and fibrosis of hair follicles and sweat and oil (sebaceous) glands.

Age-associated Losses in Skin Function and their Consequences	
Function	Consequences
Diminished barrier	More rapid and extensive entry of certain irritants or allergens.
Diminished cell replacement	Slow wound healing; weak scars.
Diminished chemical clearance	Lesser absorption of medications administered through skin.
Diminished oil production	Dry skin.
Diminished sweat production	Decreased thermal regulation.
Diminished sensory perception	Increased frequency and/or severity of skin injury.
Diminished vitamin D production	Increased risk of its deficiency, osteomalacia and bone fractures.

The nerve fibres for touch and pressure also progressively decrease to approximately one-third of their initial number, between the second and ninth decades of life. This results in diminution of touch sensation in the skin.

Subcutaneous Fat

There is usually some loss of fat beneath the skin. This deprives the older person of a useful cushion to cover the bony prominences, and it may be one of the reasons why old people are intolerant of cold and draughts.

The manner in which subcutaneous fat is distributed over the body also undergoes significant changes during the lifetime. In persons in their 60s, 70s and over, fatty depots tend to disappear from the periphery, although fat deposition is still apparent over the hips and abdomen. Most striking is the loss of subcutaneous fat from the fore-arm of an elderly person otherwise in good nutrition or even somewhat over-weight. In elderly women's breasts, there is atrophy not only of the glandular elements, but in most instances, also of the fat envelope. The loss of subcutaneous tissue in the hands, makes the veins unduly prominent. Spontaneous rupture of blood vessels leads to patches of bleeding (purpura) on the back of the hands and forearms. These are not harmful in any way though they may alarm the person.

Because subcutaneous fat is the padding that fills out and rounds the body's contours, its loss in old age, leads to an increasing sharpness of contour and a deepening of previous hollows. Bony landmarks become increasingly prominent and formerly hidden landmarks become easily visible. Typically, the tips of the vertebrae, the angles of the scapulae, the ribs, the xiphisternum, the crests and spines of the hip bone, the patella, the arch of the foot become more prominent. This contributes to the well-known bony appearance of the aged.

Stature and Posture

Many elderly persons, in addition to the bending of the trunk (kyphosis), undergo postural changes, among which slight flexion at the knees and at the hips, tends to contribute further to diminished stature.

Because the long bones do not undergo significant shortening with age, much of the loss in stature is due to shortening of the back bone, the spinal column. This results from narrowing of the disks plus loss in height of individual vertebra. Thinning of the

Old age posture

disks appears to be the major reason for shrinking stature in the middle years, and diminution in height of vertebra, is the major reason for the progressive loss in height thereafter.

The elderly are thus characterized by shortened trunks and comparatively long extremities, proportions that are the reverse of those seen in infancy and early childhood.

Bones and Joints

Throughout the middle and later years, the bones undergo a variety of changes, in which growth and regression are interwoven. Although regression of the bones (osteoporosis) may be severe, the joint (arthritic) changes dominate the picture.

The skull is unique is being free from the weight-bearing and other stresses that can cause regression of the bones. It, on the other hand, exhibits progression changes; a 2 per cent increase in circumference of the skull has been noted in 65-year olds, compared with the circumference they had at age 20.

Presence of changes in the joints such as of the knee and spine, makes it a matter of definition as a whether these should be considered as inevitable ageing changes or as pathological.

Mobility

The older person has less energy and is not so agile than he was in his youth. A general slowing up of movement is the rule. The gait becomes stiff and the steps tend to be short.

The reduced mobility may be due to changes in the nervous system, in the joints and in the muscles. In the nervous system, the loss of cells from the brain and spinal cord leads to a slowing and diminution of co-ordination in bodily movements. There is a greater tendency to fall.

Bone and Joint Changes with Ageing

1. Decrease in bone structure (osteoporosis).
2. Decrease in the intervertebral spaces leading to a loss of height.
3. Formation of osteophytes on vertebra.
4. Degeneration of the superficial cartilage of the weight-bearing joints.

Internal Changes

Changes occur in all the internal organs of the body, slowing down or impairing their functions. These changes may not be usually obvious and be seen only when the body is under physical and mental stress, as for example, happens in the case of heart, lung and kidney functions. Or they may be ordinarily obvious, as for example, the functioning of the brain and other parts of the nervous system.

Gastro-intestinal Tract

Ageing is associated with changes in function in almost all aspects of the gastro-intestinal tract. Altered motility of the oesophagus, atrophy of stomach mucosa with resultant reduction in acid secretion and constipation are just some of the changes that are commonly seen in the elderly.

Liver

The weight of the liver decreases after the age of 50, and that has been correlated at autopsy with a diminished number of liver cells. Increase in fibrous tissue is also seen. The drug metabolizing (break-down) capacity of the liver is decreased.

The levels of liver enzymes change only a little with ageing. In healthy elderly persons, standard liver function tests such as bilirubin, transaminase, hepatic alkaline phsophatase are within normal limits. Deviation cannot be attributed to the ageing process *per se* and implies the presence of a disorder.

Effect of Age on the Gastro-intestinal Tract	
Location	Changes
Mouth	Loss of taste buds and so diminished sense of taste. Decreased salivary secretion. Loss of teeth.
Oesophagus	Heart burn (reflux oesophagitis).
Stomach	Reduction in acid secretion and delayed stomach emptying, and so diminished appetite.
Small intestine	Impaired absorption.
Large intestine	Constipation.

The liver in older people has diminished regenerative capacity.

Pancreas

Normal pancreatic structure is found in only a small percentage of elderly people. Cell fibrosis and fatty changes are frequent. These changes however, are not reflected in the functions of the gland.

The calibre of the pancreatic ducts progressively increases with advancing age. The duct that dilates with ageing retains its uniform tapering appearance with smooth margins, in contrast to the sudden and irregular duct dilatation seen in pancreatic carcinoma (cancer).

The pancreas may be displaced inferiorly.

Cardio-vascular System

As one ages, arterial stiffening causes systolic blood pressure to increase and the left ventricle thickens to a similar degree in an apparently adaptive manner. However, the cardiac output (blood pushed through the heart in one beat) is not ordinarily altered by the ageing process.

Lungs

Changes occur in the lungs and the chest wall with advancing age. On opening the chest at autopsy (after death), the lungs of an elderly individual, collapse more slowly than in the younger one. This is because of the rupture and loss of elasticity of the walls of the alveoli. Total surface area of the alveoli is also diminished for gas exchange.

Age-related Changes in the Cardio-vascular System

Anatomic

1. Increased left ventricular wall thickness and increased cardiac mass.
2. Calcification (deposition of calcium) of aortic valve.
3. Decrease in the number of cells that conduct the electrical impulse of the heart.
4. Thickening of the wall of medium-sized arteries.
5. Atherosclerotic changes (narrowing of the vessels).

Physiological

1. Increase in basal systolic blood pressure.
2. Increase in basal diastolic blood pressure.
3. Prolonged contraction phase of the ventricles.
4. Prolonged contraction phase of the auricles.
5. No change in cardiac output (the quantity of blood that goes out of heart at each beat).

The more proximal bronchi remain unchanged with age except for some calcification of cartilage, but more distal bronchioles (smaller bronchi), e.g., less than 2 mm decrease in diameter.

Progressive calcification of costal cartilages (the parts that connect front ribs with the sternum) and bending of the chest (kypho-scoliosis) lead to a stiffness in the chest wall and limit thoracic expansion. Front to back diameter of the chest increases, the appearance labelled as 'barrel-shaped chest'.

Further limitation of chest expansion occurs with decreased respiratory muscle strength.

All these changes lead to early feeling of breathlessness on physical exertion and exercise.

Age-related Changes in the Lungs

1. Decrease in elasticity of lung tissue.
2. Decrease in gas exchange in the lungs.
3. Decrease in strength of respiratory muscles.
4. Increase in rigidity of thoracic cage.
5. Breathlessness on physical exertion (exertional dyspnoea).

There is also a relative decrease in coughing response to an irritant stimulus. The result is a weakened defense against excess mucus secretion and aspiration. This contributes to respiratory infection.

Kidneys

The kidneys undergo changes in structure and function with advancing age. Some changes occur in the blood vessels; others in the kidney substance proper (nephrons). In the vast majority of otherwise healthy older people, the progressive loss of kidney (renal) mass and function, is of little significance, causing neither signs nor symptoms.

Age-related Changes in Kidney Function
1. Kidneys decrease approximately 20 per cent in size by age 70.
2. Number of glomeruli (first part of the nephron) decreases by 30-50 per cent by age 70.
3. Kidney blood flow decreases by 50 per cent.
4. Decrease occurs in urine concentrating ability.
5. Creatinine clearance (an indication of removal of waste products from the blood) declines approximately 30 per cent from the fourth to eighth decade of life.
6. Decrease occurs in the ability to maintain acid-base equilibrium in the blood.

Despite the above-stated changes, there are no signs or symptoms of a kidney function abnormality in a healthy old man.

Nervous System

The size and weight of the brain diminishes with age. Shrinkage of the brain within the skull leads to widening of brain sulci, an increase in the size of ventricles and cisterns.

The nerve cells (neurons) loss begins much earlier, from the 20s onward, with a total loss of about 30 per cent by age 80. Of considerable importance are the regional variations. There is greater loss in some areas such as the superior temporal gyrus, the precentral gyrus and the inferior temporal gyrus. A total cell loss of 40 to 50 per cent over the life span has been estimated in different cortex areas. In contrast, the brain stem nuclei, show no loss over the life span.

Age-related Changes in the Nervous System Examination
1.   Irregular pupils of the eyes. 2.   Sluggish reaction of pupils of the eye to light. 3.   Poor pupillary reaction. 4.   Diminished reflex responses anywhere in the body. 5.   Diminished ankle jerks. 6.   Absent superficial abdominal reflexes. 7.   Unresponsive planter reflex. 8.   Decreased sense of pain, touch and vibration. 9.   Senile tremor.

Often people beyond 75 years do not process information as deeply as younger adults. They do not organize the information into categories as well and do not form visual images as effectively. Hence they may seem to be less intelligent in that respect.

Reproductive System

Changes occur all over in the reproductive organs in the females. In the male, they are much less marked.

Vagina. Vulvar and vaginal tissues of a women who is several years post-menopausal and who does not take oestrogen, are more or less atrophic. Shrinkage, loss of elasticity, and dryness of the vaginal mucosa (lining) are due to oestrogen hormone diminution.

Cervix. The cervix often undergoes atrophic changes. These are, to some extent, reversible with oestrogen therapy.

Uterus. The uterus undergoes retrogressive changes and becomes small and atrophic. Fibromas present in the wall of the uterus tend to atrophy, although they still cause problems.

Ovary. The ovary is atrophic in the post-menopausal period.

Breast. Loss of subcutaneous fat and atrophy of the organ occurs.

Sexuality. Sexual activity slowly declines throughout adult life, but seven out of ten healthy couples are still sexually active after the age of sixty and one in four after the age of seventy-five.

Alterations in sexual response associated with ageing are a result of generalised decrease in tone, strength and elasticity of tissues and lengthening of response time.

In older women, vaginal lubrication may take 3 to 5 minutes to occur, whereas in a young woman this takes only 15 to 20 seconds.

At the same level of arousal, the older woman will have a smaller volume of lubrication, but it may be adequate for intercourse.

All the four stages of response cycle (excitement, plateau, orgasm and resolution) are somewhat diminished with ageing. In the excitement phase, breasts are less engorged and the sexual flush may be absent. The clitoris enlarges normally, but there is no noticeable change in the labia majora. Vaginal lubrication is reduced. Vaginal ballooning occurs later in the plateau phase and is often less marked. Orgasms continue to occur but their duration is shorter and muscular contractions may also be less intense. Uterine spasms may render some orgasms painful. The resolution phase is rapid in elderly women and occasionally because of urethral trauma, is accompanied by a desire to urinate. Decrease in the strength of the vaginal contractions occurs with orgasm. Older women may report no diminution in the experience of pleasure or release gratification.

Sense Organ Perceptions

The functioning of all the sense organs, whether it concerns vision, hearing, taste, smell, touch or pain, diminishes in acquity. As one grows older, he slows down in his physical and mental processes; his response time increases. It is necessary for the younger people in the environment of the older to understand and to appreciate it; it can become easier and more congenial for both the groups.

Vision

Many changes occur in the eye leading to limitations in vision. Pupil size decreases. There is loss of transparency and increased thickness of the lens. These changes reduce the amount of light that reaches the retina. Partial compensation may be achieved by increased illumination. A 60-year old person requires approximately twice as much illumination as a 20-year old person. The 75-year old person requires three times as much.

Some older people develop cataract of the lens. Until surgically removed, such lens opacity produces problem with glare, leading the person to avoid the bright light that aids vision. At the same time, older people cannot adapt to darkness as well as younger ones, hence the tendency to use night lights.

Colour discrimination, particularly for the hues at the blue end of the spectrum, decreases steadily after the 20s. This is related to the tendency of the lens to yellow with increasing age; the yellowed lens serves as a filter for blue and violet.

Hearing

Some degree of hearing loss is not uncommon in the elderly, especially for high-pitched sounds. Yet it is quite common for elderly people to be able to hear female voices better than male voices! Conversational ability may not be affected, even though an older person is not able to hear the song of birds or the tick of his watch.

In later life, the deafness is usually perceptive, i.e., related to auditory nerve. Conduction deafness related to passing of sound along tissues and bones in the ear may have occurred earlier in life, with nerve deafness adding to the disability further in old age.

With each succeeding decade, there is an increase in the proportion of deaf people and men more often affected than women. Deafness is more often noticed in general than personal conversation, or at committee tables, and this causes the victim to withdraw from public work and often to become less sociable.

Many older people fail to appreciate how severe their deafness is until a late stage, by which time it may be too late to learn lip-reading or sign language. Unfortunately, when a deaf person suffers a stroke and needs rehabilitation, there is no progress until someone thinks of providing a hearing aid. An elderly person who is totally deaf and responds to all questions with a blank expression or a polite smile, may be dismissed occasionally as being mentally abnormal, even though one written question might have revealed the truth. Deafness is naturally a serious added disability when a patient is already mentally abnormal.

Smell and Taste

The sense of smell (never very acute in humans as compared with animals) deteriorates with age. An impaired sense of smell in older people is hazardous, particularly so in the kitchen.

Impaired sense of taste, however, does not seem to diminish a liking for food.

Touch and Pain

Sensitivity to touch and vibration appears to decrease with age. An older person may injure himself without feeling much of a pain.

Response Time

Slower response time appears to be largely a function of slowed central processing time for stimulus as opposed to increased peripheral nerve transmission time. The elderly are frequently described as cautious.

The importance of longer response time in older persons cannot be minimized. It is hazardous in many aspects of daily life: driving a car, crossing a street, and responding to various warning signals.

Most older people recognize that they are not as fast as they were in younger years. Younger persons who interact with older people should also be aware of this characteristic of old age.

2 Factors that influence Ageing and Life-Span

Some people look younger than their age in years, and some older. Some people have a longer life-span, but others having completed it, have died at a younger age.

What are the causes that influence ageing and the length of the life? A tremendous lot of research has been done on this topic. Everyone wants to look younger than his/her years and also to live longer. The results of some of the researches in this regard are as follows:

Heredity

In society, there are some families whose members live longer than the members of other families. The offsprings of parents who live longer, have a longer life-span; the vice-versa also holds true many a time. In this regard, it has been noticed that the longevity of the mother is even more important than that of the father. Differences in life-span are significantly smaller for twins born of the same ovum (monozygotic) than for dizygotic (two different ova). It is clear from the above that heredity plays a part in determining the longevity.

Environment

It has also been observed that all people living in certain regions of the world have a longer life-span; the opposite also holds true, i.e., all people living in certain other region of the world have shorter life-span. A study was conducted of many pairs of twins, amongst whom one of each moved away from the place of birth to a more affluent but less physically exerting society. It was found that the disease rate was more, and longevity shorter amongst the twins which moved to a newer cultural area, more affluent but less physically exerting. This shows that while heredity is an important

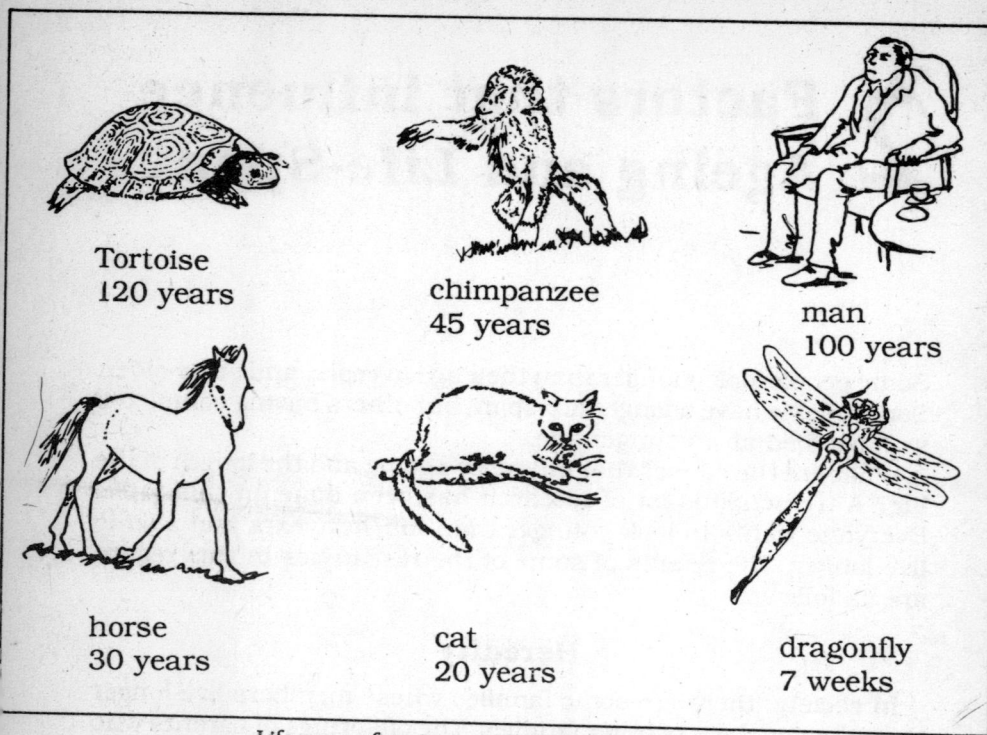

Tortoise
120 years

chimpanzee
45 years

man
100 years

horse
30 years

cat
20 years

dragonfly
7 weeks

Life span of various animals including man

factor in determining the longevity, important also are some of the environmental factors.

While we cannot decide to change our heredity, we can certainly look into the different environmental factors that influence longevity, and benefit by them.

Climate

Climate by itself, hot or cold or temperate, does not seem to have much effect on longevity. Shorter life-span of many people living in tropics seems to depend upon their relatively poor hygienic and nutritional environments.

Some studies on the tribal populations of Africa have been undertaken with regard to their life-span and the factors that could influence it. No evidence of accelerated ageing has been found in them. The two African pygmy populations, the Mbuti of North-eastern Zaire and the Babinga, were remarkably well-adjusted to the hard conditions of the rain-forest and their endurance was remarkable despite a broad spectrum of intestinal parasites. In both cases, the increase in systolic and diastolic blood pressure between 20 and 60 years of age was small, particularly in males. The serum cholesterol levels of the Mbuti were consistently low and did not increase with age.

It has been shown that the bushmen of the Kalahari desert, age in a very similar way to that of the forest pygmies. The high percentage of old people (10 per cent of the population being over 60 years of age) was also noted.

At the other extreme of the climate gradient, the Eskimos do not appear to age prematurely despite the difficult conditions under which they exert their hunting activities.

Altitude

High altitude does not appear to speed up the ageing process in individuals born and living permanently over 3,500 metres. Among Peruvian Indians, blood pressure does not increase much between 20 and 60 years of age. That altitude is not a serious handicap for resident people is also suggested by the fact that most of the highly publicised communities of 'centenarians' (Abkhascans or Hunzas in U.S.S.R.) are to be found in mountain areas.

Ionizing Radiation

People born and permanently living in areas with intense background radioactivity, like coastal Kerala in Southern India, do not appear to age more quickly than others.

There is, however, evidence available to suggest that congenital abnormalities are seen more commonly in these areas.

Air Pollution

Pollution of the environment is said to be a factor in premature ageing. This is particularly the case with air-pollution, which, as a cause of chronic pulmonary disease, might speed up the decline of lung functions normally associated with ageing.

Diet

A low caloric diet does not seem to much alter the basic pattern of development and ageing in man. The most obvious characteristic of people living on a low caloric diet is the conspicuous absence of any marked increase in body weight past their third decade of life. A low caloric diet is also generally poor in fats, particularly in saturated animal fats and has definite advantages. People living on low caloric diets, all share the privilege of having low blood pressures which do not rise with age, and low serum cholesterol which show no significant variation over the years. In most cases neither clinical evidence nor ECG indication of coronary heart disease has been found. This supports the now well documented view that the rise of blood pressure with age, so characteristic of Western societies, is a function of life style rather than an inevitable part of man's ageing process.

High caloric diets have quite opposite effects on the pattern of ageing. The most common consequence is a steady increase in weight upto 50 or 60 years of age. This rise in weight is due to a marked thickening of fat deposits with advancing age. There is also a general tendency towards a higher blood pressure rising steadily with age, high serum cholesterol showing significant increase with age upto 55 years and increased prevalence of coronary heart disease.

Some of the primitive tribal people have also been found to live on fat-rich diet. Although the daily caloric intake of the Masai, nomadic herdsmen of East Africa, averages only 3,000 calories, 66 per cent of its caloric value is made of animal fat. They take milk, sometimes supplemented with blood and meat. Their estimated average daily cholesterol intake ranges from 600 to 2,000 mg. per adult person, well in excess of the usually recommended. These people undertake heavy physical exertion and can walk or run tens of kilometers in a day. Their physical fitness is remarkable. Masai are tall and their average body weight is low (rarely above 60 kg in adults) and they look taller because they are thin due to the thinness of their subcutaneous fat layer. Despite the high fat intake, no increase in body weight and skinfold thickness is noted between 25 and 55 years of age. Blood pressure and blood cholesterol are low and do not increase with age. There is paucity of atherosclerosis (narrowing of the blood vessels) and little evidence of coronary heart disease. Such remarkable adaptation to high fat diet has also been reported in other East African cattle tribes.

The Eskimo situation is somewhat different from that of the African tribes. Their daily caloric intake can reach 3,100 calories in some tribes, of which 35 to 66 per cent is fat and 22 to 32 per cent is animal protein. However, the meat consumed is rich in polyunsaturated fatty acids. The diet is very low in carbohydrates. In studies conducted in Alaska, skinfold thickness and blood pressure do not change with age between 20 and 54 years of age.

Predominantly vegetarian people can also have too rich a diet. This has been described in the case of the Polynesians in the Tokelau Island. The diet is a traditional one of bread-fruit, *taro*, *pulaka*, fish and coconut, with chicken and pork added on special occasions. 56 per cent of the caloric intake is made up of saturated fat, 3/4th of which are supplied by coconut; pork fat also contains short chain saturated fatty acids. Cholesterol intake is very low and dairy products are rarely consumed. There is a steady increase with age of skinfold thickness in both sexes. The mean cholesterol level rises with age and so does blood pressure. Angina pectoris and myocardial infarction are present, though their prevalence rate is smaller than that of Europeans and New Zealanders.

From the above findings, it may be concluded that weight gain from eating a fat-rich diet increases blood cholesterol and blood pressure and leads to atherosclerosis (fat deposits in the blood vessels) and consequent mortality and shortened life-span.

Another important dietary factor which undoubtedly influences ageing in man is a high salt intake. Very wide variations of salt consumption exist between cultures. The Yanomamo Indians, an unaccultured tribe inhabiting the tropical rain forest of northern Brazil and southern Venezuela, do not use salt in their diet. Their major staple consists of the plantain supplemented by irregular additions of game, fish, insects and wild plants. The tribe has no access to sodium chloride. Correlatively, the Yanomamo blood pressure does not increase after the third decade of life, but even seems to decline slightly.

The Japanese are well known for their high salt intake. They are fond of a traditional diet of rice, salted pickles, *miso* and soya sauces, which are produced from fermented beans, cereals and salt. The high salt intake has been correlated with the much higher prevalence of brain stroke among the Japanese. A chronic salt overload appears to play a major role in the high prevalence of cerebro-vascular diseases in Japan.

Physical Exercise

Many of the tribals of Africa including Masai, display remarkable physical fitness and endurance despite their high fat intake. This seems to be due to intensive physical exertion begun early in life and progressively increased during the developmental years.

Psycho-social Factors

The 'stress of life' accelerates the pace of ageing. Acculturation, i.e., the process of rapid cultural change taking place when two different cultures are brought into contact, very often alters the pattern of age changes, particularly those of the cardio-vascular system. It has been found that the most acculturated at almost all ages in both sexes, show higher cholesterol levels, greater increase in blood pressure, and rise in coronary artery disease than the less acculturated.

Psycho-social factors are not only important in acculturated groups, they play a far from negligible role in more 'stable' societies. Harsh working conditions tell upon the ageing process.

The research on variations of ageing rate according to occupation and working conditions also supports the view that ageing proceeds more rapidly in some occupations than in others. A survey undertaken some years ago on assembly-line workers with a 50-hour working week and frequent night shifts in a large automobile factory near Paris, showed how poor some of their physical and mental performances were already at 50 years of age. On the contrary, the random sample of Parisian school teachers studied in the same way, exhibited quite a different pattern. Whereas their weight, vital capacity and blood pressure varied with age in much the same way as those of the 'average' middle class Parisians, their muscular strength (hand-grip) declined more rapidly, while most of their mental performances remained far superior at every age and for both sexes. Particularly striking was the fact that the teachers lost their memory only about half as fast as the controls.

Our present knowledge of how environmental factors affect the pattern and rate of ageing in man is still inadequate. There is no doubt that climatic parameters *per se* have little influence. Diet, physical exercise and psycho-social factors are of much greater importance both in traditional and industrialized populations.

It seems likely that in the twenty-first century, the factors to guard against shortening life-span would be excessive use of assembly-line processes, robots, computers, all sorts of automobiles, less physical exertion and no lack of rich food.

Centenarians Speak

Some time ago there was an interview shown on television with a Subedar Singh. He was born in the year 1886, i.e., he was 103 years old at the time of appearing on TV. A tall wiry sardarji, he said, he got up at 2 a.m., daily, took bath with cold water and then sat for prayer (*simran*). He had usually walked all his life wherever he had to go. He ate less quantity of diet and never took tea, coffee, etc.

Even now his voice, hearing, gait were normal. He said, he liked to sing *bhajans* and *kirtans* in praise of God and he was a satisfied man.

Pointedly asked as to what was the secret of his long life, he said, "I like to work, walk, eat less, remember and praise God, and am not desirous of the things around me."

There is another person, an asthma patient coming to me since 1956. He looked old to me when I first saw him: a thinly built man of short stature. When I asked him lately what was his age, he replied that he was over 100 years old. His son brings him to the clinic in a three-wheeler auto. He walks by himself, but lately with the help of a cane to stabilize himself. His hearing, eye-sight and speech are normal. He has been an asthma patient for as long as he can remember. His disease has not been very incapacitating and since he has come under my care, he regularly needs and takes medicine.

"What is the secret of your age," I asked him. He said, "It is the will of God. I do a lot of walking and eat very little food. Whenever the call from God comes, I am ready to go."

There was a teacher of mine whom I am not naming. He lived upto 83 and was the type who 'work upto the last day'. He was systematic and very hard working. Even at his age, he could work upto 10 to 14 hours a day and beat all his students in the hours put into the daily work. His secret of long life: a purposeful living.

Whether the secret of long life is 'the will of God' or 'purposeful living', 'long walks', 'uncovetousness', some common points that I have observed in people who lived longer are: a thin built, scanty food and long walks and the attitude 'let the will of God prevail'.

I think, that in a nutshell tells the environmental factors that affect ageing and the life-span of man.

3 Theories of Ageing

Ageing has been defined in medical jargon as "a progressive loss and deterioration of physiological capabilities and functions with a decreased viability, and increased vulnerability and probability of death." Ageing processes are considered to be universal, progressive, and irreversible. What exactly are the processes that bring on ageing, is not known with certainty.

Different Theories

Many theories of ageing have been propounded. In more general terms they state that:

1) Ageing is due to the gradual utilization of certain unspecific, irreplaceable materials with which the body is endowed at birth.

2) Ageing is due to accumulation of what has been termed "the debris of life," resulting in eventual clogging of the vital processes of the body.

Ageing is due to a combination of the above two. This theory is called the 'unitary' theory.

Researches done during the last two decades and the results thereof, suggest that ageing reflects the expression of a host of processes that independently and in concert, bring about the changes we recognize as ageing. It is probable that primary ageing events occur quite early in life and that even developmental processes set the stage for the decline, and, ultimately, the death of the organism.

Different Processes

The different processes that lead to ageing are described as follows:

Limited Cell Life. Data suggest a maximum dividing (mitotic) ability for various cells of different species. This is thought by some to determine the life span of a species. Cells obtained from older persons and shorter-lived species are reported to have less potential for population doubling than cells obtained from younger persons and longer-lived species. It has been observed that physiologic function begins to decline in many tissues shortly after reproductive part of the life cycle. This decline proceeds at different rates for different tissues. Although some decline in function may be tolerated for a majority of post-pubertal years, certain cell types are more critically needed for continued survival.

Repair Theory. This theory proposes that longevity is determined by the cell's ability to repair damage that may occur to DNA of the nucleus in the cell. When ultra-violet light was used as a means to damage DNA, cells obtained from longer-lived species and younger persons had the best repair capability.

Hormonal Theory. This theory is based on the belief that various neural and hormonal functions control the process of ageing and eventual death. The gradual decline in hormonal function or in the cellular response to hormones, is thought to contribute to ageing.

Immune Theory. Normal immune functions which are protective to the body begin to decline quite early in life, in fact soon after sexual maturity. The changes that take place are due to changes in the immune cells themselves. There are many cell types involved in the immune response.

The human immune system loses competence of function with age. This is evidenced by the nearly exponential increase in incidence of infections and auto-immune diseases (in which the immune cells start killing the normal body cells) and certain cancers.

The immune theory of ageing states that immune cell ageing is the essential change and ageing of other organs follows on from this.

Information System in the Cell. The cells of the body are constantly bathed by a dynamic set of hormones in the blood that include corticosteriods, thyroid hormones, catecholamines, pituitary hormones, insulin, glucagon and many others. In addition, certain cells receive input through direct innervation by the nervous system. Because hormonal and nervous signals to target cells (cells in which they are supposed to act) are essential to the integration of body function, an age-dependent loss of this information flow could cause systemic disturbances that would, contribute to the decline of the system.

On the other hand, a given target-cell type could change with time in its diminished ability to sense the hormonal/neural environment, owing to changes intrinsic to the cell. This could result in an altered cell type that may be inappropriate to its own survival or the survival of other cells that depend on its gene products.

Furthermore, genetic information stored within the nucleus of a normal cell is compacted into an ordered structure called chromatin which contains DNA and RNA. Any age-dependent effects on the flow of genetic information from DNA to RNA could profoundly influence the functioning of cells by limiting their adaptive response to hormonal stimulation.

Conclusion

Ageing seems to start at the molecular level, proceed to the cellular level, and ultimately to involve the whole body.

4 Increasing Life-span through Different Systems of Medicine

From time immemorial, man has aspired to long life, full of youth, free of disease. Different means have been used to attain this goal: prayers, use of herbals and minerals, physical means such as exercise, Yoga, and the diet.

Some success has been achieved. The life span of man has increased and some of the diseases have been eliminated or reduced, making living healthier, more productive and more worth living.

Let us now see how the different systems of medicine prevalent in India, set out to achieve it and how much they have contributed to it. Some of the methods used have been described from the original texts.

Ayurveda

Ayurveda, the Indian system of medicine, by its very name means the "science of long life". Its concept of good health covers physical, mental, moral and spiritual aspects.

Ayurveda has always given fullest attention to prevention of disease and attaining healthy long life.

Concepts

Ayurvedic concepts on rejuvenation therapy and long life, are very elaborate and time-tested. This part of Ayurveda has been termed Rasayana.

Rasayana is one of the eight clinical specialities of classical Ayurveda. It is not only a drug therapy, but is a specialized procedure practised in the form of rejuvenative recipes, dietary regimen and special health-promoting conduct and behaviour.

Charaka Samhita categorises the methods of rejuvenation as:
(1) indoor and (2) outdoor.*

The indoor method is described as follows:

In an area resided in by princes, physicians, the twice-born communities, saintly men and men of virtuous deeds, free from alarm, salubrious, close to a city, where the necessary materials may be had, one should, having selected a good site, cause a retreat chamber to be built with its face, towards either the east or the north. It should be of the following description: high-roofed and commodious, built in three consecutive courts, furnished with narrow ventilators, thick-walled, congenial in all weathers, well-lighted, pleasing to the mind, proof against noises and other disturbing agents, not used by women, equipped with all the requisite things, and having physicians, medicines and Brahmanas ready at call.

Thereafter, during the sun's northern course in the bright half of the month, when the day (*tithi*) and the constellation are propitious and the *muhurta* and *karana* are favourable, the man seeking rejuvenation should, getting shaven, enter the retreat, having fortified himself in his resolution and purpose, full of faith and single-mindedness, having cast off all sins of the heart, cherishing goodwill for all creatures, having first worshipped the Gods and then the twice-born and having performed the circumambulation of the gods, the cows and the Brahmanas.

Therein, being cleansed with the purificatory measures and on having regained his happiness and normal strength, he should undergo the rejuvenation procedure. We shall first describe the cleansing procedure.

A person deserving rejuvenation should after he has been subjected to the sudation and oleation procedures, drink with warm water the powder of chebulic myrobalans, rock-salt, emblic myrobalans, *gur*, sweet flag, embelia, turmeric, long pepper and dry dinger, all in equal parts. After his body has thus been cleansed and he has been put on a rehabilitatory diet, he should be given to drink thin barley-gruel mixed with *ghee*, for a period of either of three nights or five days or seven days, until his intestines have been purged of all faecal accumulations.

On being satisfied that the person's bowels have been properly cleansed, the physician should administer him the rejuvenation procedure most suitable to him.

Chikitsa-sthana, Chapter I, 17-74.

One of the important preparation and procedure called Brahma rejuvenation is as follows:

Take forty *tolas* (1/2kg) each of the five groups of penta radices, a thousand fruits of chebulic myrobalans and thrice that number of fresh emblic myrobalans. The five groups, each group consisting of five roots, are as follows: (a) Ticktrefoil, Indian night-shade, painted leave uraria, yellow berried night-shade and small caltrops, constitute the first group called 'the ticktrefoil group' (b) *Bael* tree, wind killer, Indian calosanthes, white teak and wild snake gourd, constitute the second group called the'bael group'; (c) Hog's weed, the two *surpa parnis*, wild green gram and wild black gram, heart-leaved *sida* and castor oil plant, constitute the third group called 'the castor oil plant group'; (d) Jivaka, *rsabhaka, meda*, cork swallow wort and climbing asparagus, constitutes the fourth group, called 'the jivaka group'; (e) small sacrificial grass, thatch grass and paddy roots constitute the fifth group called 'the grass group'.

Of each of these five groups of penta-radices, take as instructed above and mixing them, boil the whole in ten times the quantity of water. When the decoction is boiled down to a tenth of its quantity, it should be filtered and the fluid part kept. Take now the fruits of the chebulic and emblic myrobalans, and after de-seeding, crushing them in a mortar with a pestle, throw the pulp into the decoction mentioned above.

Add to this the powder of the following, the measure of each ingredient being 16 tolas (200 gms): Indian pennywort, long pepper, kidney leaved ipomea, rushnut, nut grass, embelia, sandal wood and aloe wood, liquorice, turmeric, sweet flag, fragrant poon, the small cardamom and cinnamon. Add to this the powder of sugar-candy, measuring 4,400 *tolas* (50 kg) in weight, 512 *tolas* (6 kg) of oil and 768 *tolas* (9 kg) of *ghee*. Boil all this in a copper vessel on a low fire, taking care to see that the decoction has changed into a linctus but is not burnt. Take it down and after it has cooled, add honey to it. The measure of honey to be added is half of that of the oil and *ghee* combined. The whole linctus should be kept well-mixed in an earthen jar which has been saturated with *ghee*. It may then be administered in proper dosage and at the proper time. The dose should be such as not to interfere with the taking of the patient's meals. When the medicine has been digested, the patient should be given to eat a dish of *sastika* rice with cow's milk.

Describing the efficacy of the above prescription, *Charaka Samhita* states: "The hermits known as the Vaikhanasas and the Valakhilyas and likewise other celebrated ascetics attained immense longevity from the use of this *rasayana.* Shuffling off their decayed bodies, they secured for themselves fresh youth, freed themselves from langour, weariness and breathlessness, and were unhampered by disease, were single-minded, and endowed with intelligence, memory and strength. These mighty ascetics, practised spiritual austerities and celibacy for unending years with exceeding devotion."

A second Brahma rasayana has also been described with more or less similar constituents as the first, but it contains also the powders of gold, silver, copper, corals and iron.

Chyavana prasha is also described as a rejuvenant. It is stated that, "by its use, Chyavana, though grown very old, became young once again Intelligence, lustre, immunity from disease and longevity increase."

The second category of rejuvenation procedure described in Ayurveda is based on good conduct. *Charaka Samhita,* in this regard, says:

One who speaks the truth, who is free from anger, who abstains from alcohol and sexual congress, hurts no one, avoids over-strain, is tranquil of heart, fair spoken, is devoted to repetition of holy chants and to cleanliness, is endowed with understanding, given to alms-giving, diligent in spiritual endeavour, delights in reverencing the gods, cows, Brahmanas, teachers, seniors and elders, is attached to non-violence, and is always compassionate, moderate, and balanced in his waking and sleeping, is given to regular taking of milk and *ghee,* is conversant with the effect of different weathers, season and dosage, is versed in propriety, devoid of egotism, blameless of conduct, given to wholesome eating, spiritual in temperament and attached to elders and men who are believers and self-controlled and devoted to spiritual texts; such a one should be known as enjoying the benefits of rejuvenation therapy constantly.

The above description of rejuvenation, according to Ayurveda, takes care of both the preventive and promotional use of medicinals, and psycho-social and moral aspects, all of which are being highlighted now through researches in modern medicine. These and similar other methods are bound to produce desirable effects.

Naturopathy

Naturopathy's way to long life is through cooperating with the nature to do its job well. The primary cause of all diseases, according to Naturopathy, is conscious or unconscious violation of Nature's laws. This may be in thinking, breathing, eating, drinking, dressing, working, resting, as well as in moral, social and sexual conduct.

Concepts

Disease in reality is a self-purifying effort on the part of Nature. Lindlahr states: "Every acute disease is the result of the cleansing and healing effect of Nature. If you suppress the acute conditions by drugs or by any other means, you are simply laying the foundation for chronic diseases. All diseases from a simple cold to skin eruptions, diarrhoea, fever, etc., represent Nature's effort to remove from the system some of the morbid matter, some poison dangerous to health and life."

In India, our religious texts like the Vedas and Upanishads, and the secular ones like those of Ayurveda, lay the greatest stress on living with the Nature and making use of natural stimuli for promotion of health, longevity and cure of disease.

In recent times, Gandhiji was one of the greatest enthusiasts of Nature cure methods.

Naturopathy procedures accomplish this aim by assisting Nature in removing from the body the accumulated waste products. They stimulate the organs of elimination to better functioning and thus restore the diseased and disordered organs their normal tone, blood supply, glandular activity, etc. They also intend to bring back to normal, the abnormal physical and mental habits of the patient so as to stop further harm to the body and to teach him to live with the Nature and not against it.

The procedures which naturopathy recommends to be used in maintaining and restoring health are daily cleanliness, physical exercise, relaxation and regulation of diet. They also include the use in different forms of water, earth, air and sunshine. Some people include under it measures such as massage, manipulation also.

Physical Exercise. Daily physical exercise is essential to physical and mental health. It helps in the assimilation of food that is taken and in the elimination of waste matter from the body. It tones up muscles and enhances blood circulation in all parts of the body. In India, many nature cure centres make use of Yogic *kriyas* such as *dhautis*, *netis* and *asanas* for keeping the body fit.

Diet. A well-balanced diet which contains proteins, fat, carbohydrates, vitamins and minerals in proper proportion and in quantity according to the need of the person, is essential. The food should not be, so far as possible, greatly altered from its natural state by overcooking.

Fasting. Accumulation of waste products in the body either because of over-eating or due to faulty digestion and assimilation, is considered one of the major causes of ill-health. Nothing eliminates better these waste products than fasting.

To begin with, absolute abstinence from food is recommended. After this, fruit juice in limited quantities is allowed. No hard and fast rules are set down to determine the length of the fast. Each individual case is handled according to his own needs. The foul breath, coated tongue and bad taste in the mouth are said to be the first symptoms to appear when one fasts. They are worse in those who are heavily loaded with waste products. These symptoms continue till the work of elimination is completed. A fast while it reduces weight a little, adds more to the zest and health. The good effects of fasting are enhanced by a preliminary cleaning of the bowels, which is usually carried out by an enema or bowel wash.

Use of water (Hydrotherapy). Cold water contracts the small blood vessels of the skin and produces pallor and coldness. But soon afterwards, as the cold water is withdrawn, the contracted blood vessels expand and the suffusion of the parts with an increased amount of blood, brings redness and dispels pallor. It is not the initial but the later effect of cold water, i.e., the stimulating and tonic effect that is made use of. Cold water bath is given to patients to invigorate the body and to strengthen the vital force. Gradually, as and when the patient can bear it, the temperature of the cold water is lowered further.

Application of hot water to the skin prepares the body for the application of cold. The reactive power of the body is greatly increased if the preliminary heating has taken place. In cases of fatigue, rheumatism or anaemic and enfeebled persons, this preliminary heating of the skin proves more efficacious. Hot baths also relax and soothen the body and prove effective in relieving pain. Alternate hot and cold water baths are the most stimulating.

Sun bath has been found very efficacious especially in cases of chronic diseases. In cases of debility, exposure of the uncovered body to the morning sun, acts as an all round general tonic and accelerates the metabolism.

By living with the Nature and not against it, not only one avoids disease, but also enjoys the longevity that one attains.

Yoga

Yoga is not a system of medicine, yet through it, one can attain long life and a "sound mind in a sound body."

According to Patanjali, the author of *Yoga-sutras*, Yoga, consists of eight components, viz., *yama, niyama, asana, pranayama, pratyahara, dharana, dhayana* and *samadhi*. The first four components relate more to the body; they prepare the body for the next four components which relate more to the mind.

Concepts

Yamas are the restraints: not to kill (*ahimsa*), not to lie, not to steal, not to be avaricious, and to observe abstinence.

Niyamas are disciplines like cleanliness, serenity, asceticism, etc.

The purpose of *yamas* and *niyamas* is to break the usual physical and mental habits, to make them amenable to the dictates of the will. They provide one with the capacity to think clearly and to indulge only in such activities which lead one to one's determined goal. They prevent frittering away of limited energies and time available. This helps one to feel calm and relaxed.

In order to concentrate one's mind for as long as one needs to do during Yoga practice, one must sit in a posture which is pleasant and firm. Keeping this in mind, Yoga teachers evolved and described different postures (*asanas*). According to Patanjali, an *asana* should be *sthira sukham*, i.e., stable and agreeable.

Besides the therapeutic value of different *asanas* in keeping the body fit and even in the cure of certain diseases, it has also been shown that during *asanas, pranayama* and *samadhi*, the record of electrical waves, emitted from the brain, shows a pattern that is indicative of a result relaxed state. This observation has attracted worldwide attention as mental tension and the need to lessen it, is a current major problem in most societies of the world.

Mental tension, as we have seen already, is one of the factors which lowers the resistance of the body to disease and decay.

About Yoga, our renowned sage-philosopher, Dr. S. Radhakrishnan, wrote the following even when Yoga had yet to be scientifically investigated: "In Yoga, we have all reservoirs of life to draw upon, of which we do not dream. It formulates the methods of getting at our deeper functional levels. The Yoga discipline is nothing more than the purification of the body, mind and soul and preparing them for the beatific vision. Since the life of man depends on the nature of *citta*, it is always within our reach to transform our nature by controlling our *citta*. With faith and concentration, we can even rid ourselves of our ills. The normal limits of the human vision are not the limits of the universe. There are other worlds than that which our senses reveal to us, other senses than which we share with the lower animals, other forces than those of material nature. If we have faith in the soul, then the supernatural is also a part of the natural. Most of us go through life with eyes half shut and with dull minds and heavy hearts, and even the few who have these rare moments of vision and awakening, fall back quickly into somnolence. It is good to know that the ancient thinkers required us to realise the possibilities of the soul in solitude and silence and transform the flashing and fading moments of vision into a steady light which could illumine the long years of life."

Unani Tibb

Unani medicine, also called *Tibb*, is built upon the ancient Greek medical concepts of Hippocrates and Galen as conceived and expanded by al-Razi and ibn-Sina and other Arabic and Persian physicians. It makes use of herbals, minerals and animal products to keep the body fit and to promote long life.

Concepts

Unani *tibb* postulates that every person is endowed from birth with a unique humoral constitution which represents his healthy state.

In the human body, there are four humours (*akhlat*). These are phlegm (*balgham*), blood (*khoon*), yellow bile (*safra*) and black bile (*sauda*). When these humours are present in the right proportion in the body, the body is healthy. When the proportion is disturbed, loss of health is the result thereof. In order to restore health, it is necessary to restore their balance.

Unani *tibb* also postulates of a power in the body of self-preservation. This power strives to restore any disturbance within the limits prescribed by the constitution or state of the individual. Great reliance is placed on this power, the aim of the physician being to help and develop rather than supersede or impede the action of this power.

Unani drugs intend not only to overcome the present disturbance in the body by dint of its intrinsic power but also to emerge after recovery with greater power of resistance to future disturbances.

According to Unani *tibb*, health and longevity depend upon the congenital and environmental factors, and keeping the humours (*akhlat*) of the body in equilibrium, is the secret of getting rid of any disease and attaining disease-free long life.

Homoeopathy

Homoeopathy as such does not claim to prolong life span except through treatment of disease and thereby restoring health.

Concepts

According to Hahnemann, the originator of the system, human body functions and is maintained by a vital force. This force is capable of adjusting the body and mind to the best advantage of the person when he is threatened by adverse influences. Disease means disorderly functioning of this vital force. In acute disease, this vital force though disordered to a great extent or even to the point of extinction, still retains an inherent capacity to set itself right with or without medicinal help. In chronic diseases, however, the vital force though altered in an insidious way, gets so deranged that it seems to have lost that inherent capacity of self-adjustment.

When a patient responds to treatment, according to Homoeopathic concepts, his complaints shift from one area of the body to another, usually from more vital organs to less vital organs, as if some inner healing force were directing their course. Head symptoms move down towards the trunk and gradually along the extremities to the hands and feet. Illness of vital organs such as the lungs and heart would shift into the throat or intestine, may be ending as a discharge or as a skin eruption. Mental illnesses would move into the emotional and then into the physical sphere. In the case of a long-standing disease under treatment, the most recent symptoms that the patient had, reappear for a brief period first, and the oldest symptoms, the last.

Under Homoeopathy, the symptoms of illness are often not considered dangerous in themselves to be removed by any means, but instead they represent an attempt by the body to heal itself. Behind every symptom of a particular illness is the attempt of the body to restore balance.

Living with the Nature, and using the minimum quantities of medicines, when needed, so as to reactivate the vital force of the body, brings about, according to Homoeopathy, good health, freedom from disease and consequently long life.

Tantra

Tantra makes tall claims not only for prolonging life but also for making it undecayable. These claims have, however, remained unsubstantiated.

There is a story about Nagarjuna, a great tantric of ancient times. *Katha-sarit-sagara* narrates it as follows:

"In olden times, a king named Chirayus (Long-lived) had a gifted minister called Nagarjuna, an offspring of the Boddhisattva. He knew the use of all drugs, and by making an elixir, he rendered himself and the king free from old age. One day, an infant son of Nagarjuna, whom he loved more than any of his other children, died. He was so much grief-stricken that by his force of asceticism and knowledge, he proceeded to prepare from certain ingredients, *amrita* (the water of immorality), in order to prevent mortals from dying. But while he was waiting for the auspicious moment in which to infuse a particular drug, Indra told the Ashwins, the twin physicians to gods, to go and give this message to Nagarjuna on the earth from him: "Why have you, though a minister, begun this revolutionary proceeding of making *amrita*? Are you determined now to conquer the Creator who intended created men to be subject to the law of death, since you propose to make men immortal by preparing the *amrita*. If it takes place, what difference there will be between gods and men. And the constitution of the world will be broken up, because there will be no sacrificer and no recipient of sacrifice. So, by my advice, discontinue the preparation of *amrita*, otherwise the gods will be angry and will certainly curse you. Rest assured that your son, through grief for whom you are engaged in this attempt, is now in *svarga* (heaven)."

With this message Indra dispatched the two Ashwins. They arrived at the house of Nagarjuna, and after receiving the *arghya*, told Nagarjuna, who was pleased with their visit, the message of Indra and informed him that his son was with the gods in heaven.

Nagarjuna, though despondent, yet thought: "Never mind the gods, but if I do not obey the command of Indra, these Ashwins will inflict a curse on me. I shall not proceed further with preparing this *amrita*. There is the consolation that on account of my good deeds in a former life, my son has gone to the abode of bliss."

Having thus reflected, Nagarjuna told the Ashwins: "I obey the command of Indra. I will desist from making *amrita*. If you had not come, I shall have completed the preparation of *amrita* in five days and freed the whole earth from old age and death."

After saying this, Nagarjuna buried the almost accomplished *amrita* as advised by them. Then Ashwins took leave of him and went and told Indra in heaven that their errand was accomplished, and the king of gods rejoiced.

Tantras recommend use of mercury, sulphur, their compounds and herbals for rejuvenation of the body. That they succeed in achieving their goal, has never been shown.

There is a joke which most of us have heard. I will only recapitulate it. A tantric with his disciple entered a village. He looked old and his disciples were very reverential to him. While the villagers bowed and brought them food and sweets, one among them, out of curiosity asked the disciple in a hushed voice, "What is the age of Guruji?" The disciple said, "I do not know for certain, because I have only been in his service for the last 200 years!"

Modern Medicine

Avoidance of ill-health, curing disease and thus prolonging life, has been practised through Western (now modern) medicine since the time of Hippocrates and Galen.

The seventeenth century German, Cohausen (1749), gave an account of the revitalization of old men by the breath and spirit of young virgins, in a book entitled *Hermippus redivivus, or The Sage's Triumph over Old Age and the Grave*. The book states: "Still I affirm that there are no settled periods in nature, no inevitable law, which conjoins weakness and infirmity with a certain number of years; but that is very possible, nay, and very practical too, for a man to extend the length of his life, much beyond the common date, and that without feeling the incommodities of old age, for otherwise this would rather be avoiding death than preserving life."

By the beginning of the twentieth century, it had been concluded that old age could be slowed down by an efficacious system of diet, sleep and exercise.

Animal experiments conducted so far indicate that all efficacious pharmacological therapies tested, achieve their effects by a reduction of disease vulnerability and not by a decrease of ageing rate.

Research Work

1. *Ginseng panax* widely used for years in Chinese medicine, has recently found favour in Western societies as a panacea against ageing. It has been suggested that ginseng can increase long-term resistance to stress and disease and thereby increase life-span. The active principles of the root (termed ginsenosides) are incorporated into certain drugs for old age. Substantiated reports are not available, but there is some evidence of increased arousal and adrenal response to stress in mice. No beneficial effects on life-span have been noted.

2. Professor Ana Aslan of the Bucharest Institute of Geriatrics has studied for many years the effects of procaine hydrochloride by intra-arterial injection in various disorders including peripheral vascular disease, angina pectoris, asthma and degenerative joint disease. Favourable responses in these conditions are attributed to the vasodilating and pain-relieving properties of the drug. She also observed more general beneficial effects such as improved skin texture, improved memory and an increase in both psychomotor activity and muscle strength. Procaine being not stable for long and so Gerovital H3 (GH3) was devised by the addition of benzoic acid and potassium metabisulphate. Aslan and others have found GH3 preferable to procaine hydrochloride solution. She claims a dramatic difference is mortality for elderly people treated with procaine over a 15-year period compared with controls.[1]

3. KH3 is another procaine anti-ageing drug, produced in West Germany as an alternative to GH3.[2] The basic concept of the drug is the same but the additives, including haematoporphyrin to prolong and enhance the activity of the procaine, are different. There are claims for improvement in aged persons of many of the faculties commonly impaired by ageing, viz., memory, mental concentration, sight, hearing, motor co-ordination and general emotional state. These claims have yet to be substantiated.

4. The problem of failing immuno-competence and increasing auto-immunity in older people (as already described in an earlier chapter) has been tried to be tackled by giving azathioprine and cyclophosphamide which are chemically effective in the treatment of auto-immune diseases. The results have by no means been encouraging.

An alternative approach has been to infuse immune cells from a healthy young donor into older individuals as they develop immuno-deficiency. This approach has formidable problems of ensuring a perfect immunological match between donor and host. Researches are now toying with the idea of storing immune cells in a tissue bank during youth but in preparation for old age. Then when the immune cell infusion is required, the same cells can be used.

---

1. Quoted by W. Davison in *Textbook of Geriatric Medicine*, edited by J.C. Brocklehwist, Churchill Livingstone, p. 164, 1985.
2. Ibid.

Conclusions

Making man immortal is against the laws of Nature. Good health and long-life are as much a gift of Nature as they are the results of one's own efforts of judicious planning in early life, keeping in view the role of diet, physical exercise and 'live and let live'.

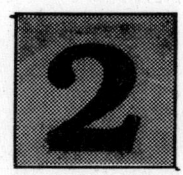

Disease in Old Age

5 Common Features of Illness in Old Age

When an older person falls ill, there are some features which are more often met because of the age and not because of a particular disease. These have to be recognized and sorted out from the particular features of a disease, so as to manage the whole patient as best as possible.

Multiple Pathology

In old age, it is a rule rather than the exception for the patient to suffer from several diseases at a time. In an acute illness, it is usually clear which disease is dominant, but some account must be taken of the others.

A patient with a brain stroke, for example, may well be handicapped also be cataract which limits his vision, heart disease which limits his capacity for effort, a urinary infection which increases the risk of incontinence, and osteo-arthritis of the hips or knees which further limits his mobility. All these as well as the stroke, demand treatment and influence his rehabilitation.

Tendency to Confusion

In an older patient, the stability of the brain is precariously balanced, probably because of the loss of nerve cells which accompany ageing. The function of the brain is readily upset by any kind of bodily disturbance, and a sudden onset of confusion is one of the commonest indications of physical illness in old age.

In a patient without previous mental impairment, the onset of confusion suggests serious physical illness, but in those whose minds are already beginning to fail, confusion may be provoked by quite minor bodily disturbances. Such reactions are often short-lived and subside as soon as the physical disorder is corrected.

Lesser Sensibility to Pain

An older patient often has a diminished sense of pain. This makes life less uncomfortable for him, but it increases the risk that he may injure himself. For example, he may burn his shins by sitting too close to the fire. Hot water bottles are a special danger.

Even serious injuries like fractures may not be obvious. An old person who breaks the neck of his femur, may have only mild discomfort even though he cannot walk.

In acute abdominal conditions such as acute appendicitis, there may be little pain or tenderness until the disease is far advanced and the patient is gravely ill.

Diminished Temperature Regulation

The regulation of body temperature is less efficient in the older patient and fever is less obvious and less severe. Thus an illness which would provoke a sharp rise in temperature in a younger patient, may in the elderly cause only a small rise or none at all.

If an old person seems unwell, there can be no reassurance in the fact that his temperature is normal. The pulse and respiration are often a better guide to his condition.

The defective temperature regulation of the older patient is also seen in his reaction to cold when his body temperature falls far below normal in the condition known as hypothermia.

Reaction to Drugs

An older patient is very sensitive to drugs, and harmful side-effects are common. Drugs are more slowly metabolized in the liver and because of diminished renal function, take longer to excrete. Thus medicines should be given in smaller doses. For example, digoxin is effective in one-quarter of the dose used for younger people. The margin of error in prescribing is less and there is only a small difference between the dose which does good and the overdose which does harm.

Moreover, one drug may react with another in unexpected ways and the multiple diseases often present, may mean that several drugs are needed. The precarious stability of the brain makes confusion a common side-effect of many drugs. Barbiturates are particularly dangerous in this respect and alternative hypnotics such as chloral hydrate and its derivatives are preferred for the older patient.

Fatigue

Persistent or recurrent fatigue is a common symptom in older patients. It is to be expected in wasting illnesses generally, but it should also suggest a search for anaemias of gradual onset. It is a prominent symptom in heart disease, in which it may be complained of as much as breathlessness (dyspnoea). It accompanies congestive heart failure, and states of low blood pressure, but in particular, left ventricular failure and cases of coronary artery disease in which the heart is enlarged and close to failing.

Sleep Disturbances

An older person's sleep is often interrupted by aches and pains of various kinds, especially rheumatic pain, the distressing ischaemic pain of peripheral vascular disease affecting the feet and legs, leg cramps, and above all, by the need to urinate at night. The latter is not uncommon even in the absence of bladder or kidney disease or diabetes.

Most insomnia is a consequence of various discomforts. In the presence of anxiety, there is usually some difficulty in falling asleep at night; with depression, the tendency is for the patient to wake early and to toss and turn. Both these disorders are common in elderly people.

Loss of Appetite (Anorexia)

If the illness is of a toxic or pyrexial nature, old patients lose their appetite completely and are content to exist for days or weeks on fluids only. Appetite is probably the last thing to recover too.

Breathlessness (Dyspnoea)

Breathlessness may be due to disorders of the lungs, heart, blood and others. An older patient may have periodic respiration (cheyne-stokes) wherein he stops breathing at all for some seconds, before resuming normal rhythm. This may appear very alarming to the attendants.

Vertigo

A complaint of giddiness or dizziness is one of the commonest symptoms among the elderly. These are subjective sensations that are always unpleasant and sometimes frightening. They indicate instability of posture, some immediate spatial disorientation, and in severe forms a sensation of rotation and extreme distress.

There are innumerable possible causes, including a simple syncopal tendency, severe progressive anaemia, gastro-intestinal bleeding, postural hypotension, hypertension, changes of heart beat (cardiac rhythm), heart attact and minor cerebro-vascular insufficiency. More localized causes are wax in the ears, acute inflammation in the inner ear (acute labyrinthitis and paroxysmal labyrinthine vertigo, Meniere's disease). The latter is fairly common in elderly patients, causing them most urgent distress as they cling to their beds in an agony of rotational vertigo, nausea and vomiting.

One particular cause of giddiness can quickly be remedied: the over-energetic use of drugs. Salicylates and quinidine in high dosage are notorious in this respect; so are even normal doses of barbiturates and anti-hypertensive drugs. Barbiturates are generally unsuitable hypnotics for the elderly, often causing considerable mental confusion, nocturnal giddiness and falls. Anti-hypertensive drug therapy is often more distressing and attended by more risk than the hypertension it is used for.

Fainting Fits

Simple syncope occurs in older people. It may be due to a sudden fall in blood pressure, to anaemia and diminished available oxygen to the brain.

The sudden loss or disturbance of consciousness may result from hyper-extension of the neck because the vertebral vessels, already atheromatous and tortuous, have been temporarily occluded in their bony canals. This may explain why some elderly patients fall dramatically when they reach up to high shelves or climb onto high chairs to shut upper windows.

Another form of attack is a hypoglycaemic episode (less sugar in blood). Spontaneous hypoglycaemia occurs even in old age, but in most cases, it takes place during the treatment of diabetes. True, the diabetes of old age is usually mild and readily controlled, but the elders are unreliable in the matter of dieting, and their appetites are fickle. They are often forgetful and muddled and the physician may be faced with a patient who is in a hypoglycaemic attack, although there is no evidence that he is diabetic. A blood glucose estimation is warranted, the more so because the state of unrelieved hypoglycaemia is so liable to precipitate heart attack or brain stroke in these patients. Oral anti-diabetic agents are particularly helpful to the elderly diabetic who cannot administer insulin to himself, but such patients are often unexpectedly sensitive to these drugs, which are capable of producing hypoglycaemic coma as insulin does.

Sudden attacks of cardiovascular causation are very common in old people. Some of them precipitate a sudden drop in blood pressure. Some may have done so, and yet the blood pressure has returned to normal only a few minutes later.

So, fainting fits, and falling may be evidence of heart attack without pain, attacks of paroxyomal atrial tachycardia, a paroxysmal fibrillation, Adams-Stokes attacks, etc. Twenty-four hour electrocardiographic monitoring of the pulse may reveal the correct diagnosis.

6 Special Hazards of Illness in Old Age

Young people get over their illness because of ample bodily reserves which help them to fight their illness. Older people have fewer reserves and so run the risk of particular complications of their illness that are not usually expected in younger individuals. Thus, a young person may be immobilized for long periods without coming to any harm, but an older person deteriorates fast in general mobility and capability, in vigour and even in spirit if he cannot move about. This happens more so in those who are already arthritic or have disorders of mobility.

Confinement to bed for older people is a harbinger of a bagful of problems. Those commonly seen are constipation, incontinence of urine and faeces, pressure sores, contractures of the joints and thrombo-embolism.

Constipation

Constipation is a common consequence of immobility or confinement to bed. It may become so severe and persistent that it is relieved only by regular enemas or manual removal. In a small proportion of cases, actual lower bowel obstruction may take place, and surgery must be used to relieve it. Many more develop faecal impaction at the rectum, which causes pain and distress, incontinent leaking of matter through the sphincter, or more commonly a form of spurious mucus diarrhoea owing to prolonged irritation of the mucosa by a large immovable faecal mass. This may additionally precipitate urinary incontinence.

Many mentally confused elderly patients disregard or are unaware of the natural demands of a distended rectum and become chronically constipated.

The fact of chronic constipation may be missed in elderly patients, especially those confined to bed, until the doctor palpates the abdomen and feels a faecal-filled colon.

Incontinence of Faeces or Urine

An old bed-ridden person may be so debilitated and inert that he is unable to exert muscular effort to control the anal sphincter voluntarily. Thus, the whole rectum is full of soft, unformed faecal matter that is neither properly retained nor properly voided.

However, the most common local cause of faecal incontinence is gross constipation. Hard masses cause impaction of the anal canal, and there is overflow incontinence of formed stool. Or faecal impaction may be accompanied by a type of mucus diarrhoea owing to irritation of the mucosa by hard faecal masses.

In older patients, rectal examination is so rewarding as to be worth making it a routine check. There is a large group of elderly patients who are incontinent both of faeces and urine because of disturbed consciousness (stupor or coma), or who lack normal brain control because of physical or vascular brain damage or established dementia. They need all the nursing care.

Pressure Sores

Any one lying in bed for long is a potential candidate for pressure sores, but an elderly patient is more prone to them than most.

The predisposing factors are many. Sensory deficit from traumatic paraplegia typically puts its victim at immediate risk because no warning of the danger comes from his own nervous system. This also applies to any elderly patient who is in coma or stupor or is totally inert or just too confused to heed the warnings from his sore skin. Additional factors are obesity, anaemia, abnormally low blood pressure, peripheral circulatory problems and faulty nutrition, either in a general respect or occasionally because of therapeutic dietary restrictions, as in a case of a low protein diet ordered because of renal failure, which can cause major tissue breakdown overnight at a pressure point. The use of sedatives in the elderly inhibits spontaneous movements. Incontinence of urine increases the risk of sores by a factor of five.

Unrelieved pressure is the overriding cause of sores. The greatest risk is when a high proportion of the body weight is applied through a small skin area, particularly where a bony prominence is close beneath the skin. The most common site is the sacrum (lower backbone), followed by the greater trochanter of the femur (thigh bone), but the heel and lateral malleolus (prominence) of the foot are often involved.

Unrelieved pressure on skin and underlying tissues deprives them of blood supply, and tissue death soon threatens.

To prevent sores, pressure must be regularly relieved and some activity in the patient encouraged despite other considerations. There are remarkably few illnesses in the elderly in which some sitting in a chair cannot be allowed. If bed rest is obligatory, the patient must be turned regularly from side to side and back to side as appropriate.

It is better to lose a little sleep than the integrity of the skin and to be turned is often a welcome relief. The vulnerable areas must be kept clean and dry and gently massaged with powder.

Thrombo-embolism

Thrombosis of deep leg veins is liable to occur in elderly immobile patients.

Calf tenderness may or may not be present and swelling may not be apparent. Unilateral leg swelling is highly suspect, particularly so in a heart patient. There is a very high death rate from pulmonary embolism (blockage of a lung blood vessel) in the older age-group and there is great difficulty in distinguishing the condition clinically from heart attack.

So great is the hazard from deep vein thrombosis in the immobile elderly, that all efforts must be made to prevent it. Patients with paralysis of the legs must have regular passive movements of both limbs. Regular inspection and measurement of the girth of the leg are as important as inspection of the pressure areas.

Death from pulmonary embolism in a bed-ridden patient is not uncommon, but must be avoided.

Contractures

Contractures are more or less fixed deformities of joints that result from their being held immobile, usually in unsatisfactory positions. Sometimes this is the result of pain, because of which the patient tries to get the joint into the most comfortable position regardless of the effect of this on subsequent function. A patient suffering from rheumatoid arthritis is particularly prone to it.

In a contracture, fibrosis of the structures around the joint (periarticular) takes place. The associated muscles become weak and shorter, often causing their tendons to be as tight as bow-strings, across the angle of the contracture. So much so that bony bridging across the joint space may take place in time.

It usually takes time for the contractures to develop. Lying curled up in bed for hours and days together allows time for the joints to get fixed in the posture in which they are held. Sometimes however, the contractures develop in a matter of two or three days even.

Brain strokes account for many contractures at the wrist, shoulder and fingers and also for many instances of foot drop. Bed-ridden demented patients sometimes have bizarre contractures because of the posture which they adopt for sitting. Patients having paralysis of the lower limbs develop planter-flexed fixity of the ankles, even when there is no neurologic deficit. This is due to the pressure of the clothes on the limbs which the patient can neither move nor feel.

The commonest contracture in the elderly is at the knee joint, with secondary flexion at the hip or vice versa.

Once a contracture is established, it may be necessary to excise the fibrous structures, lengthen short tendons. Good results can be obtained by encasing the limb, extended as far as possible, in plaster of Paris, and waiting for some days.

Contracture prevention is vital because treatment is difficult and sometimes risky and painful.

7 Drug Administration in Old Age

Ageing causes changes in the body with regard to drug absorption, distribution and action. It is important to understand this changed behaviour of the body towards drugs so that a proper response is obtained, and side-effects eliminated or diminished.

Factors Influencing Drug Response

Absorption. Following their absorption, all drugs pass in the portal (abdominal) circulation to the liver where some undergo substantial metabolism before entering the general circulation, a phenomenon known as the first-pass effect. A reduction in liver metabolic activity is likely to be reflected in a reduced first-pass effect and increased systemic bioavailability following oral administration of the drug.

Distribution. The age-related decline of serum albumin concentration produces significant increase in unbound plasma concentration of several drugs that are strongly bound to protein (e.g., salicylates, sulfadiazine and phenylbutazone). The adverse effects of corticosteroids occur more frequently in patients with low serum albumin concentrations.

Metabolism. The enzyme system in the liver is the major site of drug metabolism. There is an overall tendency for the metabolic activity of the older individuals to be less efficient than in the youth.

Excretion. For some drugs, e.g., antibiotics like streptomycin, and digoxin, the kidney is the major route of elimination. Changes in renal function associated with ageing have important implications for such drugs. The elderly are at risk of reduced clearance and resulting accumulation of the parent drug and the active metabolites.

Action Response. Response of the body to drugs depends on their action on target tissues and organs. This ultimately reflects the ability of the free or unbound concentration of the drug to react with specific cell or its parts, and to initiate specific action. That action is modified by factors such as homeostatic control mechanisms, the influence of disease states, and concurrent medications.

There is increasing evidence that age may alter responsiveness to drugs. Isoprenaline infusion produces less increase in heart rate in older patients than in younger individuals.

Patients with liver disease are more likely to experience adverse neurologic effects of cimetidine, a drug used in cases of stomach ulcer. This is related to an apparent change in blood-brain barrier to cimetidine in the presence of liver disease.

The above aspects have to be duly taken care of while prescribing drugs in the elderly people.

Profile of Patient Liable to Adverse Reaction to Drugs

1. Small elderly female.
2. History of allergic illness.
3. Previous adverse reaction.
4. Multiple chronic illnesses.
5. Renal and mental failure.

Practical Considerations

Older people suffer illnesses more often than do the younger ones, and they may suffer from more than one disease at a time. Hence, they need to take drugs more often and at a time for more than one disease. As a result, there is more likelihood of side-effects of the drugs being witnessed. Greater care is thus needed in the administration of the drugs in the elderly.

**Considerations Recommended
while Prescribing Drugs in the Elderly**

1. Individualize medication dosage. Start low, go slow.
2. Determine blood levels wherever possible.
3. Not all elderly can tolerate 'therapeutic levels' usually prescribed.
4. Side-effects well tolerated during youth may not be tolerated during older age. For example, orthostatic hypotension on standing has greater potential for inducing stroke, heart attack and/or renal failure because of more common predisposing factors.
5. Medication interactions and side-effects become additive and even synergistic as the number of medications being

taken increases. Hence limit the number of medications taken whenever possible.

6. Choose the form of medication most easily administered.
7. All medications should be clearly labelled.
8. Instruct the patient what to expect from a medication and what to do if the desired effect is not achieved.
9. Keep dosage schedules as simple as possible.
10. Carefully consider efficacy versus side-effects.

The elderly have special difficulties. Forgetfulness may lead to poor compliance, with the potential of either under-dosing or over-dosing. Failing vision, small print on medication lables, and ambiguity of tablet size or colour, make it relatively easy for the elderly patient to err in taking tablets as directed. Such errors may be compounded by the common practice of mixing medications in a single container.

If possible, the physician should include the indication in the instructions for labeling, such as 'for blood pressure', 'sleeping pill', 'for arthritis', so that the patient and relatives can recognize the proposed role of medication.

Major Problems Encountered with Medication Use in the Elderly

1. Reduced compliance.
2. Drug-drug interactions.
3. Drug-nutrient interactions.
4. Side-effects, often poorly tolerated.
5. Paradoxical response may result from a given medication.

Patients should be encouraged to dispose of medications that are no longer being used to avoid possible confusion with necessary medication at a later date.

A simple chart of medications and the times at which they are to be taken, can be helpful.

Is the Drug Really Needed?

With increasing number of older patients and with increasing diagnosis of common disorders such as hypertension and old age (maturity-onset) diabetes, it is critical that we optimize our therapeutic strategies. There is little doubt that elevated blood pressure and blood glucose levels contribute to morbidity and mortality in all age-groups. However, the evidence is far from clear that the normalization by drugs of either blood pressure or blood glucose in entirely asymptomatic patients, contributes to improved longevity, reduced morbidity or a more desirable quality of life in the older patient.

8 Guidelines for Prescribing Antibiotics in Old Age

Absorption, distribution, metabolism and excretion of antibiotics are all altered in the elderly. Thus, there is an increased incidence of adverse side-effects in this age group.

Kidney (renal) insufficiency which occurs with ageing, has a major influence on the actions of many antibiotics. Hence the elderly need to be guided if they have to take antibiotics.

Penicillins

Metabolic and neurological toxicity may occur in the elderly patient with renal function impairment, if dosages are not properly adjusted.

Many penicillins contain a large amount of sodium and must be given cautiously to the elderly patient.

Nafcillin, oxacillin, cloxacillin and dicloxacillin (all different compounds of penicillin) are only slightly affected by renal insufficiency.

Ampicillin is frequently associated with diarrhoea.

Cephalosporins

All doses of cephalosporins must be adjusted in patients with renal insufficiency except the third-generation cephalosporin, cefoperazone, which is excreted primarily by the liver. The third-generation cephalosporins, cefotaxime and moxalactam as well as the second generation cephalosporin cefuroxime cross the blood-brain barrier.

Neurotoxic reactions may occur with high doses of the cephalosporins.

Most parenteral forms contain a significant amount of sodium; all oral forms are sodium-free.

Streptomycin, Genticin

The margin between therapeutic and toxic doses is narrow especially in the elderly patient. A borderline-normal serum creatinine in an elderly patient with little muscle mass may indicate significant renal insufficiency. Renal toxicity may be prolonged and may rarely be irreversible.

Inner ear toxicity (ototoxicity) is more common in the elderly patients with renal insufficiency or preexisting hearing loss. Auditory nerve toxicity is more common when streptomycin is used with diuretics or when a patient is in renal failure. Stopping the drug may prevent further damage.

Neuromuscular paralysis is a rare but potentially serious side-effect and may be treated by prompt administration of calcium.

Clindamycin

The drug is metabolized in the liver; hepatic dysfunction may produce a five-fold increase in serum half-life. Dosage should be reduced in patients with liver disease.

Inflammation of large intestine (pseudomembranous colitis) occurs more frequently in elderly patients. Treatment consists of stopping the drug and initiating oral vancomycin (non-absorbable).

Chloramphenical

It crosses the blood-brain barrier in the presence of inflammed and normal meninges.

Dose-related anaemia results from reversible bone-marrow depression. Irreversible aplastic anaemia may occur.

It is metabolized primarily in the liver; dosage must be adjusted in hepatic insufficiency.

Erythromycin

Adverse reactions are uncommon. Jaundice may follow administration of the estolate form in 10 per cent of treated patients and is reversible on stopping that drug. The estolate salt should be avoided in older patients because of risk of liver toxicity.

Dose-related upper abdomen (epigastric) distress, nausea and vomiting are common.

Excretion is primarily in the bile and faeces. Elderly patients with slow gastrointestinal motility may have lower serum levels.

Tetracyclines

It is rarely the antibiotic of choice in the elderly. Diarrhoea is common with it. It is primarily excreted by the kidney. It may produce renal failure rapidly in patients with preexisting renal insufficiency.

Demeclocycline may cause skin lesions on exposure to light (phototoxic dermatitis).

Inner ear function of balancing the body (vestibular reactions) may be disturbed, especially with minocycline.

Liver toxicity may occur following parenteral route with normal doses in patients with renal insufficiency.

Trimethoprim-Sulphamethoxazole (Septran)

Adverse reactions are more frequent in females, but not related to age. Nausea, vomiting and rarely diarrhoea may occur. If skin rash occurs, the drug should be stopped.

Elderly patients with low serum folate levels, i.e., cases of malnutrition, malabsorption, alcoholism, are at risk of developing blood toxicity. Folic acid administration is indicated in this situation. Strictly speaking, this drug is not an antibiotic. But it is widely used in older patients.

9 Management of Nutritional Problems in Old Age

Malnutrition is common among the elderly. This is because of many and varied causes, some of which are as follows:

Factors Involved in the Development of Malnutrition in the Elderly

1. *Physical impairments*
   Poor vision
   Poor dentition/dentures
   Arthritis
   Immobility
2. *Physiological impairment*
   Malabsorption and maldigestion of food
   Loss of taste and smell
3. *Pathological conditions*
   Dementia
   Depression
   Disease states such as cancer, parkinsonism, hypothyroidism, atherosclerosis.
4. *Social factors*
   Poverty
   Alcoholism
   Poor dietary habits
   Isolation
5. *Treatment-related causes*
   Drug nutrient interaction
   Prescribed diets

Oral Diet
The older patients are not only the largest users of drugs, they also

continue using them for longer periods because of the chronic nature of their diseases. There is a likelihood that some of the drugs they take, may interfere with absorption of some of the nutrients in the diet and lead to their deficiencies. This is particularly so because many older people already take less quantity of diet and have self-imposed restrictions on their diet.

Potential Drug-nutrient Interactions	
Drug	Nutrient Deficiencies
Mineral oil	Vitamin A, D, K, E
Phenolphthalein	Potassium, Vitamin D, Calcium
Colchicine	Fat, Vitamin B_{12}, Potassium
Phenformin	Vitamin B_{12}
Glucocorticoids	Calcium, Potassium
Antacids	Phosphate
Potassium chloride	Vitamin B_{12}
Aspirin	Iron
Diphenylhydantoin	Vitamin D, Calcium
Furosemide	Calcium, Potassium, Magnesium, Zinc, Water, Sodium
Isoniazid	Vitamin B_6
Warfarin	Vitamin K

Some of the special diets prescribed by the doctors to their patients suffering from particular diseases, are also liable to lead on to malnutrition if continued on for longer periods.

Special Diets with Potential for Adverse Effects	
Special Diet	Potential Problems
Lactose-free diet	Suboptimal calcium intake, subsequent osteoporosis.
Low-protein diet	May lead to protein malnutrition with hypoalbuminemia and muscle wasting.
Low-salt diet	Food apathy and decreased nutrient intake secondary to lack of taste.
High-fibre diet	Bloating; gas and/or abdominal distension.

Recognition of nutritional insufficiency is more complicated in the elderly because of numerous age-related changes in body composition and physiology. However, history of the patient, particularly of the details of the diet and the drugs that he takes, coupled with the signs and symptoms, do help in coming to a conclusion.

The underlying disease should be properly assessed so that there is improved digestion and absorption, as for example, hypothyroidism, parkinsonism, cancer.

Nausea because of a special diet or drug should be corrected and other oral and dental problems should be managed.

Constipation is one of the common problems in the elderly. Its elimination should be sought, so far as possible, through natural means. Giving of more fibrous foods is one such means. A diet high in fibre may reduce constipation as well as alleviate some of the symptoms of the irritable bowel syndrome. Fibre holds water, resulting in bulkier and often softer bowel movements. Although there is no definitive recommendation for fibre intake requirements, and intake of approximately 20 gm a day is probably safe and adequate for most healthy individuals. This can be achieved either by diet or with supplements.

Approximate Fibre Content of Selected Foods (gms/100gm of the material)

Grains and cereals		Green beans	3.2
White bread	2.7	Corn on cob	4.7
Whole wheat bread	8.5	Cauliflower	1.8
Corn flakes	11.0	Broccoli	4.1
White rice	0.8	Baked potato	2.5
		Baked beans	7.3
Fruits		Lettuce	1.5
Prunes	7.7	Cucumber	0.4
Banana	3.4	Onions	2.1
Raisins	6.8	Carrots	2.9
Apple (peel and flesh)	1.5	Celery	1.8
Cherries	1.2		
Dried apricots	24.0	*Others*	
Orange	2.0	Peanuts	8.1
		Peanut butter	7.6
Vegetables		Lentil soup	2.2
Peas	12.0	Strawberry jam	1.1
Spinach	6.3		

Tube (Enteral) Diet

Older patients who cannot swallow food either because of general weakness or due to difficulty in swallowing (dysphagia), have to be provided food by stomach tube, so as to maintain their nutrition.

The initiation of tube feeding should only follow a complete assessment to determine that the patient is receiving an inadequate oral intake. Patients with marked weight loss and/or clinical or laboratory signs of protein-calorie malnutrition, almost always should be supplemented, particularly if those factors that led to the malnourished state are not readily reversible.

Small, soft polyurethane tubes specifically designed for feeding should be used. These tubes permit continued oral intake. By placing the tube distal to the pylorus, the risk of pulmonary aspiration is minimal.

A wide variety of nutritionally complete, commercially prepared enteral supplements are available to suit almost any patient.

Medical Conditions Commonly Requiring Tube (Enteral) Nutritional Support

1. Neurological/psychiatric diseases
   Cerebrovascular accidents
   Cancer
   Trauma
   Severe depression
   Anorexia
2. Oropharyngeal/oesophageal
   Obstruction
   Cancer
   Dysmotility (derangement of movements in the oesophagus)
3. Gastro-intestinal disorders
   Mild to moderate malabsorption
   Inflammatory bowel disease
   Fistulas (connective opening of bowels with other abdominal organs)
4. Adjunct to medical/surgical treatments
   Burns
   Chemotherapy
   Radiotherapy

The enteral route should be considered first in patients with a functional gastro-intestinal tract because of ease of administration, low cost, proven long-term efficacy, and good patient tolerance.

Parenteral (Intravenous)

A variety of situations frequently encountered may preclude adequate oral or tube feeding.

Indications for Intravenous Nutritional Support
1. Bowel obstruction 2. Coma 3. Some bowel fistulas 4. Intractable vomiting 5. Impaired swallowing mechanism 6. Severe malabsorption with or without diarrhoea 7. Tetanus 8. Jaw, wired and closed as in trauma cases

Depending on the severity and likely course of the underlying disease that precludes oral intake and the nutritional status of the patient, parenteral nutritional support may be indicated. It should be considered in those situations in which maintenance or improvement in nutritional status allows for significant improvement of the underlying illness or permits proper therapy to be administered, or recovery to occur.

10 Surgery in Old Age

Three types of situations arise in the elderly with regard to surgery.

First, where there is no choice and the surgery has to be done as an emergency, as for example, in cases of intestinal obstruction.

Second, where the operation has to be done, but it is not an emergency, as for example, prostate removal. Here there is time to plan an operation and if there are some risk factors in the patient, they can be corrected or improved upon.

Third, is the type of situation where there is some controversy whether a surgical operation should be done or not, as for example, coronary by-pass surgery for angina pectoris. In cases of controversy about surgery, the important thing to keep in mind is, whether the patient would not be worse after it, in so far as looking after himself independently.

Emergency surgery in older people, carries a far greater mortality and complications after the operation. This is particularly so if the patient is suffering from heart disease, diabetes, renal and liver disorders.

Risk Factors Management

If the surgical operation is not an emergency, the risk factors present in a particular patient can be assessed and steps taken to minimize their significance.

Careful preparation leads to safer surgery. An old person's physiological reserves are diminished and the stress of an operation tests him to the full. Surgery is often complicated by failure in a system other than that in which the surgeon is operating and in the majority of elderly patients, there are also medical problems which demand consideration.

Cardiovascular. A patient in heart failure requires diuretics and digoxin. An old person who has had a recent heart attack (cardiac infarction), should, if possible, have his operation postponed for three months. A patient with ischaemic changes as seen in his ECG, runs a risk of further coronary trouble after surgery.

The cerebral circulation also requires consideration. If there is evidence of cerebrovascular insufficiency, operations may be avoided if possible, as there is some risk of stroke.

The veins too are important. Thrombophlebitis and pulmonary embolism are among the common complications of surgery. A history of previous thrombophlebitis may give a warning.

Respiratory. The greatest hazard of all after surgery is bronchopneumonia. Many old people have bronchitis and a period of treatment with an antibiotic combined with breathing exercises and postural drainage can be of great value. The surgical risk is much reduced if the patient gives up smoking.

Attention must be given also to the hygiene of the mouth. Any carious dental stump should be removed. This reduces the risk that the patient will inhale infected material after operation.

Common pulmonary complications such as of respiratory insufficiency, pneumonia, lung collapse (atelectasis), occur more often in patients with pre-existing chronic lung disease.

Kidneys and Bladder. Operation should be avoided until renal failure has been corrected. The patient should be asked about his bladder function, as incontinence following surgery is common. In men, prostate is examined as retention of urine is a well known complication after any operation.

Bowels. Old people are prone to constipation and faecal impaction is common. No patient should go to the operation theatre with a loaded rectum.

Diabetes. The older patient with diabetes will do better if carefully stabilized.

Drugs. Certain drugs have to be increased before the operation, e.g., corticosteroids.

Psychological. The surgeon needs to assess the patient's personality and morale. Anything which can allay his anxiety and depression will be of help.

Mobility. Immobility predisposes to pressure sores, so steps need to be taken to make the patient walk as soon as possible.

Nutrition. Obese people are more liable to the complications of surgery. If there is time for the patient to lose some weight, he/she may do so.

If there is severe anaemia, a blood transfusion would be necessary.

Cardiac Surgery

It remains an area of controversy. Even though cardiac surgery carries a greater risk for the elderly, the risk/potential benefit ratio must be carefully evaluated in order to make the therapeutic choice. Age should never be used as the sole determinant of surgical risk. Other factors, such as general medical condition and presence or absence of pre-existing severe cardiac disease, must be considered. Each case must be individualized. Coronary artery by-pass surgery continues to remain an area of controversy. Recent data suggest that although the perioperative cardiac complication rate (5-10%) is higher in the elderly, continued medical management of left main or three-vessel coronary artery disease may result in an even higher mortality rate.

Making Anaesthesia Safer

All anaesthetic drugs depress cellular function to a greater or lesser extent. Suitable combination of them and techniques have to be chosen to limit unwanted depression of cellular function, particularly in the brain, heart, liver and kidneys. These considerations assume special importance when the surgery is stressful or associated with significant blood loss or tissue trauma.

11 Home and Hospital Care

Care of an elderly person either at home or in the hospital is not an easy matter. He needs to be protected from physical injury. More importantly, he needs to be protected from mental injury which he may suffer due to unintentional, but sometimes intentional fault of others around him.

Safety in the Home

More accidents to the elderly happen inside the home than outside. The great majority result from falls, but a number of them are from burns. Some of these disasters can be avoided by better planning. The most dangerous places are the stairs, the kitchen and the bathroom. Many falls occur around the bed.

Stairs. The staircase should be well lit and equipped with a handrail. A loose mat should never be placed at the foot or the head of the stairs, and nothing should ever be left on them.

Kitchen. Kitchen storage cupboards should not be too high. No one should have to stand on a chair to reach them. The oven operated by electricity or gas should stand at table height. Many old people find it difficult to stoop down to a low oven. If they lose their balance while holding a hot dish with both hands, they cannot save themselves and risk burns as well as a fall.

Bathroom. An old person feels safer if there is a handrail fixed in the bathroom.

The lavatory also needs appropriately placed handrails and for some people a raised lavatory seat is an advantage.

Mental Tension

For older people who have once enjoyed a position of authority, it is never easy to step down into a subsidiary role. They can remain content only if they feel loved and appreciated and if their position

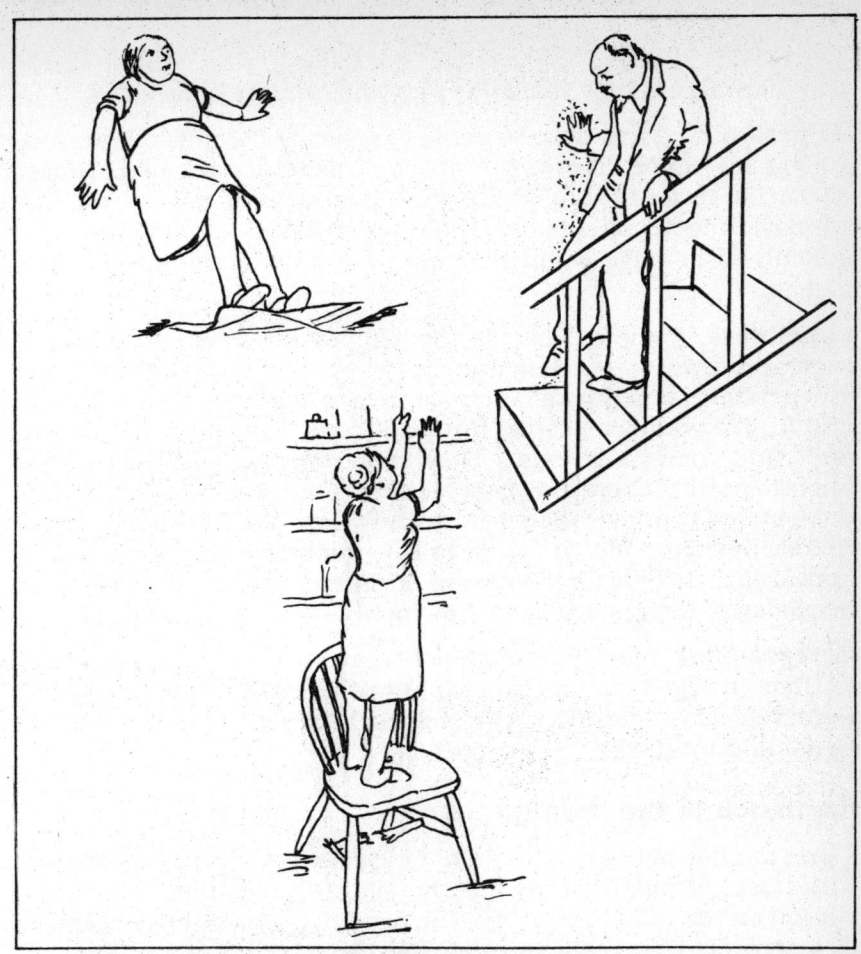

Situations where one can fall

and security within the family is assured. Old people need to be needed and this is easier if they can be of some service, however small, to others.

Failure to achieve this adjustment is a potent cause of tension within the family. In his fear of losing status and authority, the old person may be driven consciously or unconsciously to 'difficult' behaviour. He makes unreasonable demands upon his family and in this way becomes his own worst enemy. Conversely, a member of the younger generation may refuse to play a subordinate relationship role to his parents and this too produces stress.

The tensions between an old person, who cannot accept an

appropriate role and the younger generation, who cannot make him feel valued, may make life very difficult for both sides.

Rejection. Matters usually come to a head when an old person suffers an acute illness, the onset of incontinence or perhaps nocturnal restlessness. Where an old person is ill or very frail, his admission to hospital is nearly always required. He may be more difficult to manage when he comes back home after the acute illness.

Loneliness. Some old people throughout life have antagonized their relatives and neighbours. They may be aggressively independent, repelling all offers of help. They may be very lonely and unlike younger people, find it difficult to make new friends and find new interests. They may become nervous and apprehensive. Others may become depressed and apathetic. They do not usually parade their grief in any dramatic way but withdraw themselves from life. They fail to eat properly, to attend to their appearance, to care for their home. This is likely to lead to physical breakdown, depressive illness or mental deterioration.

Bereavement. Most people after bereavement, gradually adjust to their changed circumstances, but others are unable to do so. Bereaved old people, like younger ones, have problems, emotional, social and financial.

Admission in the Hospital

There are few patients who do not experience significant anxiety with hospitalization. Many elderly regard the hospital as a way-station on the road to eternity. The need to go to the hospital may be interpreted, correctly or otherwise, as evidence of a serious or worsening disorder. With most hospitalized older patients, one can correctly assume fears of dying and death.

Hospitalization may produce a reactive depression or increase the depth of a preexisting one. A person reduced to semi-helplessness, either by his illness or the hospital environment may react profoundly to the loss of usual relationships. This combined with weakness, helplessness and feelings of isolation, often leads to depression.

12 Rehabilitation

Rehabilitation is the process whereby the patient is helped to regain the greatest possible degree of personal independence. It is a matter of team work and involves all those who have any dealing with the patient. By working closer together, the team generates an atmosphere of activity and optimism which is the hallmark of a good team.

Rehabilitation seeks to improve the motor performance of the disabled elderly so that he can attain or maintain his pre-disease functional status. The techniques that are employed are essentially symptomatic because the chronic diseases of old age are usually degenerative and incurable. The goals of rehabilitation are to reduce the limitations imposed by these impairments and to prevent the consequences of disease.

The techniques employed make use of heat, cold, massage, electrotherapy, hydrotherapy and ultraviolet radiation. Occupational therapy and braces, splints and prostheses are also used to enhance function.

These techniques are prescribed for the following indications: relief of pain, increase in range of motion, increase in motor power, increase in skill and increase in endurance. The approach to management depends on the etiology underlying the symptom.

Relief of Pain

Heat is a valuable agent in providing pain relief in musculo-skeletal disorders of the aged, such as those due to rheumatic diseases. It may be given to superficial structures by a hot-water bag, paraffin bath, or an infrared lamp, and to deep structures by diathermy, microwave or ultrasound machine. Heat is contra-indicated locally in the presence of occlusive vascular disease, in which increased tissue metabolism cannot be met by increased blood flow. It is also contra-indicated in the presence of cancer. When there is acute inflammation involving a nonexpansible area such as bursitis, heat may exacerbate the pain.

Intermittent cold packs (ice) may then be useful as an analgesic. In some patients with exquisitely painful musculo-skeletal disorders such as low back pain or even pain of nerve compression, cold may provide symptomatic relief.

The application of heat and cold to elderly patients should be carried out with full awareness of all the considerations which are of less consequence when younger persons are treated. The elderly often have diminished perception of heat and cold. Without the protection of normal sensation, they may be subjected to the risk of trauma from these modalities. Occlusive vascular disease may compound the injury. It is often present without a history of intermittent claudication, because the inactive elderly person may not walk long enough to develop typical symptoms.

Thermo-regulatory mechanism may be impaired in the elderly. Hence care has to be taken to see that prolonged exposure to body heating may result in high fever (hyperpyrexia), and exposure to cold may result in hypothermia.

Increase in Range of Motion

The elderly tend to develop contractures relatively quickly if they are bedridden for some time or in a wheelchair for most of the day or if a body part is immobilized by a cast. Thus immobilization of a body part should be as short as possible.

Range of motion of a joint may be increased by the use of passive exercises or stretching. Stretching should be accomplished only by a physical therapist or other trained person to avoid trauma and aggravation of underlying disease.

Increase in Motor Power

Ageing is associated with a decrease in strength, speed and coordination.

Increase in motor power is obtained by active exercise. Passive exercise, no matter how prolonged, does not effect strength. Active exercises produce increased strength in the muscles. Isotonic exercises encourage full ranged of motion of joints and counteract the restrictive effects of immobilization.

In elderly persons, isometric exercises should be avoided as they put undue load on the heart.

Increase in Skill

When a person limps, the energy cost of walking is much higher than the cost of normal gait. Repititive exercises tend to improve motor skill by improving the efficiency with which a given task is performed. Improvement in skill may also be obtained by the use of assistive devices, braces, and canes.

Increase in Endurance

Isotonic exercises have a training effect on the cardiovascular system and the heart itself. Such exercises may lead to an increase in endurance, that is, the length of time or the number of times that an activity can be carried out. Isotonic exercises train both skeletal and heart muscle and may produce changes in the oxygen transport system. The muscle cell enzymes increase, which thereby cause economy in the use of oxygen. Other changes may include a greater arteriovenous oxygen difference and a marked increase in the number of capillaries supplying a given area of muscle tissue. In addition, there is evidence of a training effect on the heart muscle (myocardium) itself, so that the resting pulse rate may diminish and stroke volume may increase. Obviously, any exercise that the elderly carry out should be aerobic, with a steady rate easily attained and therefore submaximal, with avoidance of any oxygen debt. One simple technique for monitoring the elderly during any exercise activity is the pulse rate. Particular attention is paid to the elderly patient whose resting pulse is above 100 or whose immediate post-exercise pulse exceeds 120. A pulse rate over 130 is often indicative of excessive stress and could lead to dire consequences.

Prognosis

There are some guide-lines to help in predicting recovery from chronic disability such as that produced by stroke. In general, as with many neurologic disorders of brain, spinal cord or peripheral nerves, the earlier the return of function appears, the greater the return that takes place. For example, if there has been no significant return of function in a flail arm and hand, one month after a stroke, they are likely to remain non-functional.

Incontinence of bladder and bowel that persists in a stroke patient for more than several days, is a poor prognostic sign. Bowel incontinence of central origin usually signifies a severe defect. Left hemiplegia (paralysis) is often associated with a poorer outcome than right hemiplegia. The left hemiplegic even though he usually has no language disorder, often shows poor judgment, disturbance in abstract thought and perceptual motor disorders. These characteristics interfere with carrying out the tasks of daily life, and they may subject the patient to undue risks of trauma.

Chronologic age *per se* is not closely correlated with successful outcome in rehabilitation. Physiologic age is often the more significant determinant. For example, a man of 75 with the same amputation as a 55-year-old man may suffer less severe disability if he is thinner, if he had been athletic as an adult, in contrast to sedentary habits in the younger man, and if he has no other significant health problem such as cardiac disease or arthritis, which could be found in the 55-year-old man.

Concomitant disabilities may also influence the outcome. For example, if the amputee needs to use one or two canes, but has rheumatoid arthritis in his wrists, his capacity to walk would be seriously compromised because he would need his arms for assisting in his walk. Finally, the *sine qua non* for success is either the patient's motivation or an environment that influences him to attain feasible goals.

13 Social Responsibility for the Elderly

Older people have always occupied a position of respect in Indian homes and in social life. Because of their experience and wisdom, they can guide and help the younger generation.

There is an interesting story in this regard. A boy of a village fell in love with a girl of another village. The girl's people were not in favour of their marriage, but did not like to say No directly. They said that they have some conditions which if fulfilled, only then could the marriage take place. They directed the boy to, "Bring twenty youngmen of your village in the marriage party but no old man."

The boy's people agreed but nevertheless took an old man with them hidden in a big fruit basket. On arrival, the boy's people were told that each of them would be served a cooked goat and if each one could finish his goat in one sitting, then the marriage will take place.

The boy's people were perplexed because they were not sure whether each of them could finish off a complete goat. In their perplexity, they silently consulted the old man. He advised them to ask the bride's people not to serve twenty goats at once, but one goat at a time to be divided among the twenty people; only after the first goat was finished, was the second to be served, till the last. The bride's people could find no excuse for it, and started serving.

Lo and behold! After a short interval, all the goats were eaten up and they departed with the bride.

The moral of the story is that the old man from his experience and wisdom guided the younger people so that they could achieve their goal happily.

The older people are needed in the home and the society in which they live because of their experience. The older people also need the company and care from the younger people, because of the infirmities imposed upon them by their old age. While the parents of children are busy in their domestic and social roles, the grandparents keep company with the grandchildren.

But the picture has changed in the Western world and it is changing in the East too. In India also, the smaller nuclear families have no place for old people, so that the older people feel lost and uncared for. When they fall ill, there are no special facilities available to them, as happens in the West. They have to compete for treatment and hospital beds with the other patients who being younger, more often have only incidental diseases from which they recover, while the older patients with their degenerative and chronic diseases hardly manage to come out of the hospitals, and hence find difficult to get a bed.

With the increasing population of older people in India as well, some organizations are coming up to cater to the needs of the older patients, so as to provide them medical assistance in its diverse forms.

Help-Age India

Help-Age India is one such organization which is doing a commendable job in this direction. Its aims and objectives are:

—To foster the welfare of the aged in India, especially the needy aged;

—To raise funds for projects which assist the elderly irrespective of caste or creed;

—To create in younger generation and in society, a social awareness about the problems of the elderly in India today.

It is a registered national voluntary organisation dedicated to improving the quality of life of the elderly in need of help. With its headquarters in Delhi, it operates throughout the country. Since its inception in 1978, it has provided about Rs. 87.6 millions to help set up 523 projects for the welfare of the elderly. Most of the funds were raised within India. It is dependent on public support for the continuation of its work for the care of the elderly.

Help-Age India also provides training to sponsored candidates for the care of the old.

A Mobile Medicare Unit visits older people in the villages and examines them, and provides medicines and other facilities wherever necessary.

Help-Age India is linked to the growing worldwide movement of concern for the elderly through its membership of Help-Age International. As one of the first national units to come into being in a developing country, Help-Age India consultants have given advice and guidance to other developing countries to set up their units.

14 Preventive Health Care in Old Age

Prevention of disease is a better proposition than cure in any age group. It is much more so in the elderly, because while children and adults may easily recover from a disease, the older patients do so tardily and sometimes only partially. Hence prevention of disease in them carries a much greater significance.

Care about prevention of disease in the older patients can be taken at three different stages:
(1) Primary, i.e., to prevent illness to take root and to maintain optimal health,
(2) Secondary, i.e., to detect disease at early stages, and to cure it as soon as possible, and
(3) Tertiary, to prevent further progression and complications of the disease.

Primary Prevention

This means taking care about the dos and don'ts of health so that the person maintains good health and does not fall ill. The following measures are important in this regard:

Adequate Nutritional Intake. In general, a protein intake of 0.8 gm/kg body weight is sufficient to maintain a positive nitrogen balance. Failure to do so increases the risk of infection and fatty infilteration of the liver, etc.

Intake of refined glucose should be limited. These foods are low in vitamin and fibre content, and increase risk of dental caries. Carbohydrates should comprise 50 to 60 per cent of most diets.

Saturated to unsaturated fat ratio should approximate 1:3 and total fat intake should be limited to not more than 20 per cent of calories.

A well-balanced diet consisting of at least 1500 to 2000 calories should provide under most circumstances adequate intake of vitamins and minerals. Although sodium intake should be minimized, recent data suggest that only a minority of elderly are "salt-sensitive". In general, sodium intake should not exceed 5 gm/day.

Elderly persons rarely require supplemental iron.

1200 to 1500 mg of elemental calcium is the daily recommended requirement.

Since many elderly do not consume a diet high enough in calcium, oral supplementation may be necessary.

A well-balanced diet should contain the required 15 mg of zinc which has been shown to be essential to wound healing. Sources of dietary zinc include meat, chicken and fish.

Adequate fluid intake is essential to maintain normal renal and bowel function.

Adequate fibre helps guard against constipation, piles (haemorrhoids). Fibre must be introduced in the diet slowly so as to avoid intestinal symptoms and poor compliance.

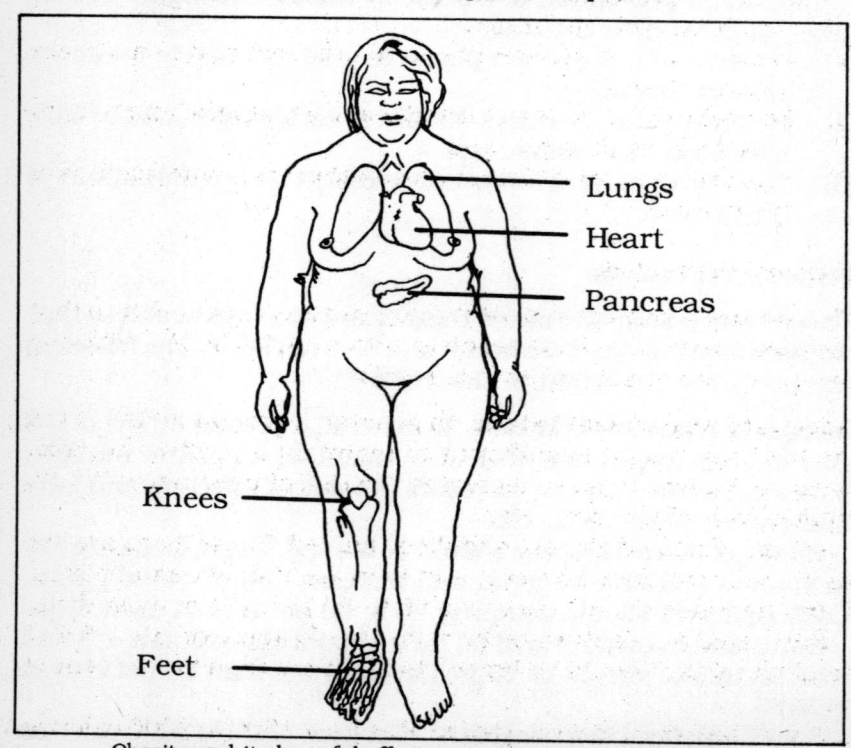

Obesity and its harmful effects on various parts of the body

Avoid Over-weight. With increasing age, the weight should decrease rather than increase. A weight more than 15 per cent of what it normally should be, is a health hazard. Over-weight predisposes to osteoarthritis, diabetes, hypertension and makes a person accident-prone.

Stop Smoking. Smoking increases the risk of getting chronic bronchitis, emphysema and chronic airway obstruction. It increases the risk of getting lung cancer. More frequent upper respiratory tract infections occur in the smokers.

Smoking also increases the risk of getting coronary artery disease and the heart attacks. Hence smoking should be stopped.

Avoid Alcohol. Changes in body composition that occur with age result in decreased extra- and intra-cellular fluid compartments. The same intake of alcohol in the elderly as during youth, may now result in a higher effective alcohol level increasing the risk of falls, depression and mental disturbances.

The onset of alcoholism is a major problem in the elderly, particularly in men who have recently lost their spouses. Hence alcohol should be avoided.

Physical Exercise: Physical exercise is capable of retarding loss of bone mass, improving cardio-pulmonary function, improving mobility and benefitting the psychological profile.

Exercise programmes should include isotonic exercises wherein the tone of the muscles remains the same as for example jogging. These consist of full muscle movement without resistance. This is in contrast to isometric exercises wherein the muscle length remains the same, as for example, weight lifting. In the latter, the muscles work against force. These result in excessive increase in peripheral vascular resistance and raised blood pressure. Isometric exercises are not recommended and should be avoided.

Exercise should begin gradually and increased slowly.

Suggested Guidelines for an Exercise Programme in the Elderly
1. In the beginning, the patient may be discouraged by an increased amount of muscle and joint soreness. This is to be expected, and the patient should probably start with a more gradual regimen.
2. Patients should avoid eating substantial amounts of food for approximately 2 hours before and 1 hours after exercise.

3. Elderly patients have often less ability to adapt to temperature extremes. Hence care should be taken in warm climates to guard against dehydration. In cold climates care should be taken against hypothermia by wearing proper clothing. The intensity of exercise should be decreased with climatic extremes.
4. All exercise sessions should be preceded with a gradual warm-up period and terminated with a full cool-down period.
5. Care should be taken not to take excessively hot showers or baths, since this can sometimes be deleterious to cardiac function and may precipitate a syncopal episode.
6. When ill, patients should refrain from exercising.
7. Patients should know when to stop exercising: unusual discomfort, shortness of breath, chest pain or palpitation require immediate exercise termination and medical consultation.
8. Exercise should be done in safe, well-lighted flat surface.

Psycho-social Needs. A comprehensive preventive health care programme must insure that all psycho-social needs are met.

Financial security is necessary to insure adequate nutrition, shelter and medical care.

A social network including family, friends and colleagues is essential to optimal functioning.

A safe, barrier-free environment should be established. Environmental hazards can include loose rugs, inadequate lighting, stairs and inappropriately placed electric cords and appliances.

Periodic Health Evaluation. A yearly comprehensive medical evaluation is recommended for all healthy persons over the age of 60 years. The evaluation should include a thorough history and physical examination.

Secondary Prevention

In order to detect disease or a tendency to setting in of a disease and to take measures to cure it, a thorough physical and laboratory check up is necessary.

The physical check up should include the following:
1. Evaluate height, weight and skin-fold thickness.

2.   Evaluate vision, hearing, and oral, pharynx status.

3.   Monitor blood pressure, evaluate for orthostatic hypotension, peripheral vascular disease and heart.

4.   Examine breasts of both men and women.

5.   Prostate should be examined for size and for masses.

6.   A pelvic examination is necessary.

7.   Observe for signs of contractures, posture and muscular weakness.

8.   Assess for neuropathy, gait disturbance and coordination.

9.   Palpate thyroid gland and evaluate for signs of hyper or hypothyroidism.

    The following laboratory tests are also recommended to be done:

     Haemoglobin, TLC, DLC

     Blood glucose

     Blood urea nitrogen and creatinine

     Liver function tests

     Cholesterol and albumin

     Thyroid function tests

     ECG

     Chest X-ray

     Urinalysis

     Stool examination for occult blood

     Mammogram

     Cervical Pap-smear

Tertiary Prevention

This involves preventing progression of the disease and its complications. This applies to most of the chronic diseases from which the older people suffer, such as hypertension, diabetes, kidney, lung, liver and nervous system disorders, etc.

The steps to be taken, in regard to them have been detailed in Part Three of the book.

3

Specific Diseases

15 Digestive Disorders

Eating is a pleasure with most older people. Disorders that interfere with it, cause them much distress.

Diseases of the digestive system are common in the elderly. Normal ageing is also associated with alteration in the function of almost all aspects of digestion and absorption. Loose or lost teeth and diseased gums interfere with eating. Transport of food from the mouth to the stomach through oesophagus may be a painful process. Stomach may have ulcers which it has carried along with it from youth and middle age, or there may be cancer. Flatulence and constipation are perpetual problems in order people because of a variety of factors such as diminished mobility, lesser disgestive power of the enzymes, change in food habits, anxieties, etc.

Organs associated with gastro-intestinal tract, such as the liver, gall gladder and the pancreas. which normally help in digestion and absorption of food, suffer from various disorders which may be inflammatory in nature or malignant.

Acute inflammation of any of the organs in the abdomen, many a time, presents with features different from what they are in youth, and are thus difficult to diagnose and so more hazardous.

Oral Cavity

Oral problems are the commonest among the elderly. They include the problems of the teeth, the gums and the jaws.

TEETH

Loss of some or all the teeth occurs commonly in old age. Changes in the structure of the existing teeth also occur. Some of these changes are as follows.

Attrition

It is the wear and tear of the substance of the teeth more

particularly of the upper surfaces. It may be so much as to cause loss of tooth substance even to the level of the gums.

Cause(s). They are many, and more than one may be working in a patient:

1.   Attrition is greatly enhanced by night grinding.
2.   Abrasive foods produce accelerated wear and loss of tooth height.
3.   Production of less saliva (xerostomia) also contributes to dental attrition in the aged.
4.   It may be greately enhanced by envor011mental conditions, associated with some occupations such as of masons, stone-workers and carpenters, etc.
5.   Faulty or over-zealous tooth brushing, coarsely abrasive dentifrices used on hard bristled brush.
6.   Acids from citrus fruits and soft drinks. Lime juice in warm or hot water is more acidic than orange juice and its enamel-decalcifying effect is enhanced by warming.

Treatment. It is to avoid the above-stated causes as far as possible.

Dental Caries

It is a very common disorder in the elderly.

Cause(s). It is primarily attributed to the germ streptococcus mutans.

Treatment. Poor oral hygiene mainly arising from the difficulty of removing plaques from the denuded roots of the teeth, should be corrected.

GUMS

There is a high incidence of advanced gum disease in the aged.

Infections (Pyorrhoea)

Breakdown of the tooth-supporting structures is responsible for more oral disease and loss of teeth than any other disorder in the elderly. As one advances in age, the gums are attached more to the root of the teeth than to their main body. The gums recede more and more, exposing the teeth as well as their roots. This slow exposure of the roots does not result *per se* in loss of teeth, but when the additive effect of infection due to faulty hygiene is super-imposed, the effect upon the integrity of the teeth is ruinous.

Cause(s). Many causes combine together to damage the gums.

Causes of Gum Disease in the Elderly

A. Local

1. Plaque formation.
2. Food impaction and retention.
3. Rotting of food particles in the spaces between the adjacent teeth.
4. Excessively soft and sticky consistency of diet.
5. Mouth-breathing.
6. Poor cleaning of the mouth after eating.
7. Tooth mal-alignment.

B. Systemic

1. Post-menopausal osteoporosis.
2. Protein-deficient diet.
3. Vitamin-deficient diet.
4. Diabetes mellitus.
5. Other debilitating diseases.
6. Taking of drugs such as phenytoin.
7. Dryness of the mouth which may be drug-induced.

Treatment. Any of the above operating in a case should be removed.

MUCOUS MEMBRANE

Mucous lining of the mouth in older people is thinner, pale and dry. There is less blood flowing through it. If it is injured, it heals slowly.

Infections and Cancer

Cause(s). Diabetes in the old aggravates any disease in the mouth, particularly the infections. Gum and root abscesses about the teeth are common and suddenly take a turn for the worse. Any old person having frequent occurence of infections should be investigated for diabetes.

The lips and lining of the mouth are liable to cancerous change in those who smoke pipes and cigars and cigarettes.

Treatment. Use of tabacco in smoking and chewing should be stopped.

Oesophagus

Oesophagus is a tube-like structure in the neck and thorax that connects the end of the mouth (pharynx or oral cavity) with the stomach situated in the abdomen below the diaphragm.

Common disorders of the oesophagus in the elderly are: (1) Difficulty in swallowing (dysphagia), and (2) Hiatus hernia.

Dysphagia

It presents as difficulty in swallowing, initially with solid foods and later with semi-solid or even liquids. Patients complain that the food seems to "stick on the way down."

Cause(s). It may be due to any of the following causes in the oesophagus:

1.   Inflammation.
2.   Constriction of the lumen due to the presence of cancer.
3.   Disorder of the oesophageal muscles, as occurs in myasthenia gravis.
4.   Disorder of the nerves, as occurs in brain-stem palsy.
5.   Anxiety neurosis.

Treatment. The cause should be removed, surgically or otherwise.

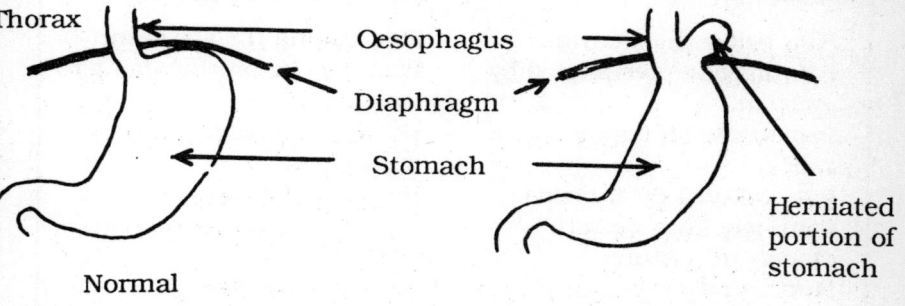

Thorax

Oesophagus

Diaphragm

Stomach

Herniated portion of stomach

Normal

Hiatus hernia

Hiatus Hernia

As the oesophagus passes through the diaphragm from the thorax into the abdomen, sometimes an actual space gets created around this opening. Whenever the pressure in or on the abdomen increases, some of the abdominal contents, mostly the stomach, can slide through this space (hiatus) into the thorax.

Cause(s). The occurrence of hiatus hernia increases with age because of the loss of strength in the muscle fibres of the diaphragm. Over-eating, smoking, and obesity can also hasten its occurrence.

There may be no symptoms when the hernia is mild and infrequent. Symptoms occur because of the: (1) entry of the abdominal parts into the thorax, and also (2) entry of acidic contents of the stomach into the oesophagus.

Heartburn is a specific symptom noticed after fatty meals, change in position such as lying down or bending to tie shoe laces, a heavy meal or tight undergarments. This results in an increased abdominal pressure exceeding that of the oesophageal sphincter. This leads to the entry of the gastric acidic juice into the oesophagus which may become inflamed, ulcerated and thus hurt.

Frequent occurrence of ulceration can cause bleeding and patient may bring out a mouthful of blood or more.

Sensation of heartburn or pain in an older person has to be differentiated from pain of coronary artery disease. The following points are very relevant in this regard:

Differentiation of Heartburn from Coronary Artery Disease

Heartburn	*Coronary artery disease*
Pain below the sternum	Pain behind the sternum.
Pain may be precipitated by emotion.	Pain may be precipitated by emotion.
Pain worse on taking tea or coffee.	No effect of tea or coffee in most cases.
Pain relieved by antacids.	No effect of antacids.
Pain may improve with change in posture.	Change in posture has no effect.
Pain usually not exacerbated by exertion.	Usually worsened by exertion.
No E.C.G. changes.	E.C.G. changes usually seen.

Treatment. Symptoms of hiatus hernia can be managed without resorting to surgery. The following preventive measures and/or precautions are necessary:

1.   Correction of obesity, i.e., weight loss to within 15 per cent of average weight for age.

2. Avoid late evening meals.
3. Avoid large meals, especially with high fat content.
4. Avoid excessive hot drinks.
5. Avoid alcohol.
6. Stop smoking.
7. Head of bed should be raised by 4 to 6 inches.
8. Avoid many pillows under the head while sleeping.
9. Avoid wearing constricting garments around the abdomen.
10. Avoid acute bending over.

If the above measures do not prove adequate, use of antacids has to be considered. Drugs such as cimetidine (Tagamet) and ranitidine (Zantac) have been found to be helpful in the treatment of hiatus hernia and heartburn.

Iron or blood transfusion will be needed if there is anaemia or bleeding (acute hemorrhage). These measures usually suffice to keep the older patient comfortable. If they fail, surgery may have to be considered.

Stomach and Duodenum

The main disorders of the stomach in elderly persons are: (1) Stomach (gastric) ulcers. (2) Stomach cancer (carcinoma).

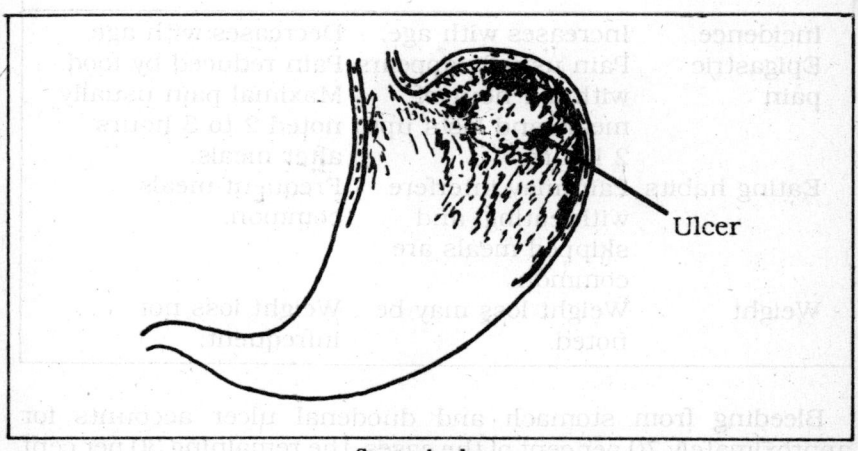

Stomach ulcer

Stomach Ulcer

It starts in old age and occurs on the lesser curvature of the stomach. It usually causes weight loss, vomiting, vague abdominal pain and occasional hemorrhage.

Cause(s). Drugs used in the treatment of joint pains which include corticosteriods and the nonsteroidal anti-inflammatory agents (e.g., aspirin, indomethacin, phenyl butazone) are known to precipitate the symptoms.

Uncharacteristic presentation of symptoms is more common in older people than in the younger. The following points may be noted in this regard:

1. Poor localisation of pain in abdomen is common. Pain may not be related to the taking of food.
2. Loss of appetite and weight may be such as to suggest a diagnosis of stomach cancer.
3. Flatulence is common.
4. Heartburn, when present, may be confused with coronary artery disease or a hiatus hernia.
5. Severe anaemia may result from chronic blood loss.

Stomach ulcer has also to be differentiated from duodenal ulcer. The latter may be present in an older person as a legacy from younger age.

Differentiation of Stomach Ulcer from Duodenal Ulcer		
	Stomach ulcer	*Duodenal ulcer*
Incidence	Increases with age.	Decreases with age.
Epigastric pain	Pain usually appears within 1 hour of meals and lasts upto 2 hours.	Pain reduced by food. Maximal pain usually noted 2 to 3 hours after meals.
Eating habits	Pain may interfere with eating, and skipped meals are common.	Frequent meals common.
Weight	Weight loss may be noted.	Weight loss not infrequent.

Bleeding from stomach and duodenal ulcer accounts for approximately 70 per cent of the cases, the remaining 30 per cent result from oesophageal varices due to cirrhosis of the liver and carcinoma of the stomach.

Diagnosis is made from the history of symptoms in a patient and physical examination. Endoscopic examination by introduction of a gastroscope into the stomach, wherein the inner lining of the stomach can be seen, helps in clinching the diagnosis. If necessary, a biopsy of the suspected area of the stomach lining can be taken to rule out the presence of cancer.

Treatment. Antacids provide some relief. Healing of the ulcers is quicker and the tendency to bleeding reduced by administration of ranitidine and cimetidine tablets. Renitidine is safer in older patients.

The patient, if under-nourished, should be encouraged to take a nourishing, mixed, well-balanced diet, in small amounts at a time.

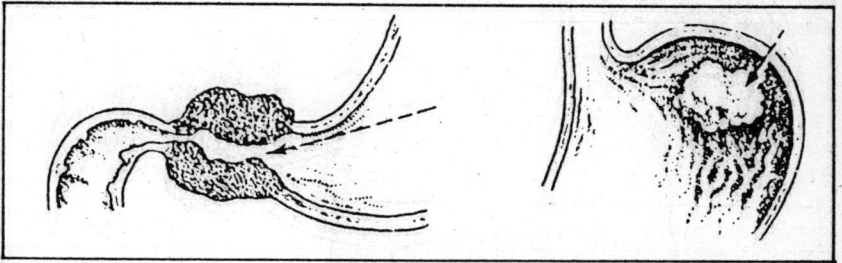

Stomach Cancer

Stomach Cancer

The symptoms may be akin to those of stomach ulcer. Loss of appetite, diminution in weight and general weakness, may be more marked.

Cause(s). These are not known with certainty.

Treatment. Diagnosis is established by endoscopic examination and biopsy of the suspected area. Many a time, the diagnosis is established late so that providing surgical cure may not be possible. Relief of some symptoms is attempted by administration of drugs.

Small Intestine

Digestion and absorption of food occurs mainly in the small intestine. Older people are prone to disorders of absorption of food and to acute obstruction.

Malabsorption

The commonest symptoms of malabsorption are lassitude, general malaise and loss of weight, anaemia, sometimes accompanied by discomfort in the abdomen. The skin may be pigmented.

Failure to absorb fat may lead to the passage of pale stools which float on the water, a condition known as steatorrhoea. The patient may complain of diarrhoea, but the abnormality of the stools is not always obvious to the naked eye. Chemical analysis, however, shows that the patient is passing more than normal amount of fat in the stool.

Cause(s). They are varied and many. The exact cause has to be found in an individual case in order to treat properly and adequately.

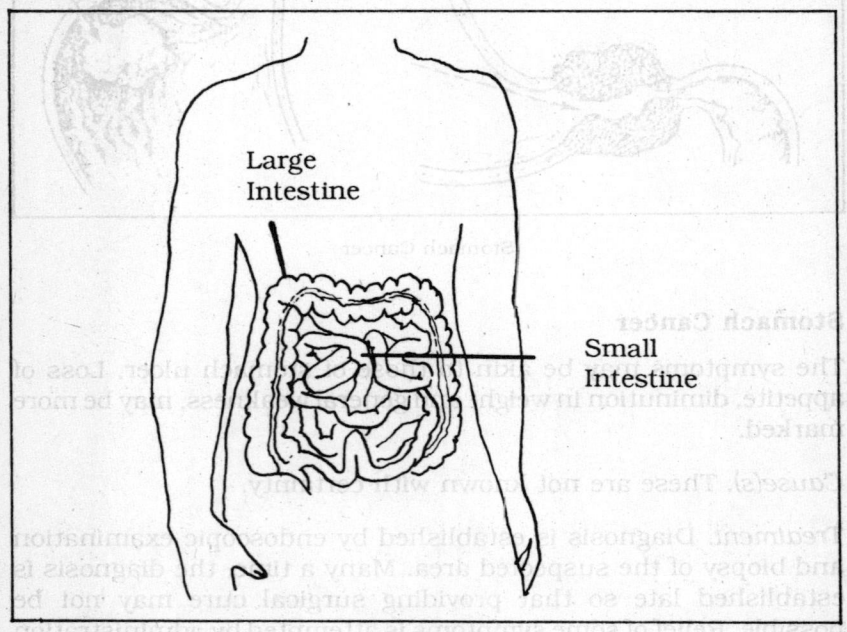

Intestines

The investigation of a patient with small intestinal disease is a complex affair requiring X-ray, biochemistry of blood, and biopsy of the small intestine.

The most important test is the collection of stool for the estimation of faecal fat. The patient takes a normal diet but no oily medicines. All the faeces is collected during the test period which may last from 3 to 5 days.

Treatment. It consists in treatment of the cause through drugs or surgery and giving of drugs and food in order to ameliorate the deficiencies already caused by malabsorption.

Large Intestine

The commonest disorder of the large intestine is constipation.

Constipation

When the contents of the small intestine enter the large intestine, they are liquid. By the time they are passed as faeces they have become solid. In their journey down the colon, much water is absorbed and their bulk is reduced by four-fifths.

The rectum is normally empty and the faeces are stored in the sigmoid colon. From time to time, the bowel propels faeces into the rectum and when this happens, a call to stool is felt. This desire can be inhibited if there is no convenient opportunity for defecation. If ignored, the desire goes away but returns later when more faeces passes into the rectum. Constipation implies the abnormal retention of faecal matter in the large bowel.

Cause(s). They are many. Delayed passage may be due to a diet with too little fluid and to little fibre. Many drugs reduce the activity of the colon; they include codeine, morphine, iron, calcium, atropine and related substances used to relieve spasm. Parkinsonism and depression also lead to constipation.

Rectal examination is the first step to detect constipation and faecal impaction.

Proctoscopy, sigmoidoscopy (which mean examination of the lowest part of the large colon) and barium enema help in finding out the cause of the condition.

Complications of Constipation
Local
Faecal impaction.
Anorectal (a little above the anus) ulceration.
Piles which may bleed.
Faecal incontinence.
Rectal prolapse (protrusion of the rectum from the anus).
General
Anaemia due to bleeding piles.

Loss of weight and weakness due to diminished appetite.
Irregular pulse and heart beat.
Aggravation of symptoms of angina pectoris.
Heart attack (myocardial infarction) in a patient having
coronary artery disease.

Treatment. Regular balanced diet containing fair amount of
roughage and green vegetables, is conducive to having normal
motions of the bowel. Physical exercise is a must for normal bowel
habits. Adequate amount of water should be taken daily. The urge
to pass stools at regular hours should not be ignored.

Laxatives when needed may be taken. Those which soften the
stool e.g., containing paraffin compounds and ispaghula husks
(Ispagol), are better than the laxatives containing magnesium salts.

Suppositories and enema are needed when there is some mild
impaction of stools.

A purgative should not be given to a patient having faecal
impaction. It is likely to cause abdominal pain and will not clear
the rectum. In such cases, it is necessary to begin with a manual
removal of scybelae. Enemas or suppositories are given daily or
on alternate days (if the patient is frail), until the bowel is seen
to be clear on rectal examination. This commonly takes a week or
longer.

Flatulence

It is abdominal discomfort due to the presence of air or gas in the
stomach or intestines.

Cause(s). It is mostly caused by excessive swallowing of air
(aerophagia). With each swallowing 2 cc. to 3 cc. of air enters the
digestive tract. Aerophagia may be a manifestation of nervous
tension or depression in the elderly patient who, having previously
been productive, is now beginning to question his/her role in
society.

If an older person is not an air-swallower, but suffers from
flatulence, he may be suffering from a digestive or absorptive
disorder of the intestine so that undigested food substances reach
the large bowel. In order people, lesser production of acidic
stomach secretions allow bacteria and parasites to live comfortably
in the bowel and produce excessive gases.

Treatment. Attention to proper chewing, swallowing and oral
hygiene and dietary alteration may have substantial effect.

Foods to be avoided include inadequately cooked starch, high fibre food, and certain legumes and vegetables, such as beans, peas, cabbage, cauliflower.

Establishment of regular bowel habits, avoidance of strong spices like red pepper, are recommended. Avoidance of stress is desirable.

Cancer of the Colon and Rectum

These are not uncommon in older people. Cancer of the colon affects both sexes equally, but cancer of the rectum is commoner in men. They present with a change in the bowel habit, either diarrhoea or constipation or else with abdominal pain due to obstruction of the large intestine. They may also cause rectal bleeding.

Cause(s). It is not known with certainty. Retention of faeces for longer periods habitually, is incriminated.

Diagnosis is established by sigmoidoscopy or proctoscopy.

Treatment. Wherever possible, it is surgical, since there is a good chance of permanent cure if operation is undertaken early. The patient may be left with a colostomy, i.e., opening of the distal colon on the abdominal wall.

Piles

Piles (haemorrhoids) cause trouble when they bleed, and when they protrude from the anus after defecation. They are not often painful unless they become strangulated which is due to thrombosis in the veins of a prolapsed pile. It causes a large purple swelling which protrudes from the anus and is difficult to reduce.

Cause(s). They are common in older people who suffer from constipation, diarrhoea or prostatic obstruction. They may accompany carcinoma of the rectum or colon.

Unless they are prolapsed, there may be nothing visible externally and proctoscopy is an essential part of the examination.

Treatment. Application of ointments or similar medications provides temporary comfort.

Piles which bleed can be treated by the injection of sclerosing solutions.

Piles which prolapse usually require to be treated surgically.

Acute Abdomen

There may be minimal symptoms pertaining to abdomen. Instead of the acute pain in abdomen, the patient may have loss of appetite, and abdominal distension. There may be no fever or only minimal. But the pulse rate and respiration rate is increased. The patient may be confused or even delirious. The doctor needs to have a high degree of suspicion in order to make a correct diagnosis. If the condition is not diagnosed early enough, the death rate is very high.

Cause(s). They are many and varied:

1. Inflammation of the gall bladder (acute cholecystitis).
2. Small bowel obstruction, due to:
   Hernia (inguinal, femoral, midline).
   Adhesions and bands from previous surgeries.
   Thrombosis of the blood supplying artery.
3. Large bowel obstruction, due to:
   Volvulus (twisting of the intestine).
   Cancer.
4. Faecal impaction of the rectum.
5. Diverticulitis (inflammation in a pouch of the intestine).
6. Pancereatitis (inflammation of the pancreas).

Quick diagnosis is needed. CT scanning may provide a clue.

Treatment. It consists in removing the cause which can mostly be done surgically. Afterwards, antibiotics are needed for treating bacterial infection, both aerobic and an-aerobic.

Liver, Gall-Bladder and Pancreas

Jaundice

Jaundice is not uncommon in older people. The yellow colour of the jaundiced patient is due to staining of the tissues with the bile pigment, bilirubin. Bilirubin is formed from haemoglobin from the red cells which have completed their life span.

The level of bilirubin in the blood rises when the breakdown of red cells is excessive, or there is disease of the liver cells, or when there is obstruction to passage of bile from the liver and in the gall bladder and its ducts.

The jaundice may be very deep, and itching of the skin is common. Bleeding (haemorrhage) may occur because of a lowered prothrombin level in the blood. The patient may experience pain when there are gallstones, but jaundice may be entirely painless. The urine is darkened by the presence of bile. The stools are pale because of its absence.

Cause(s). The common cause of jaundice in an older person is obstruction to the outflow of bile from the liver. Malignant obstruction is seen one and one-half to two times more commonly than obstruction due to the presence of a stone. Carcinoma of the head of the pancreas is the most commonly encountered cause of malignant biliary obstruction, followed by metastatic deposits from the lung, stomach, colon, gall bladder, kidney, breast and prostate.

Another cause of jaundice in the elderly is drug-induced hepatitis. Drugs that may adversely affect the liver are allopurinol, many non-steroidal anti-inflammatory agents (ibuprofen, naproxen, indomethacin, phenylbutazone), anaesthetic agents such as halothane, antibiotics, erythromycin, nitrofurantoin, penicillin, sulfonamide, antineoplastic agents (azathioprine, 6-mercaptopurine, methotrexate), isoniazid, rifampicin, methyldropa, procainamide, quinidine, chlorpropamide, tolbutamide.

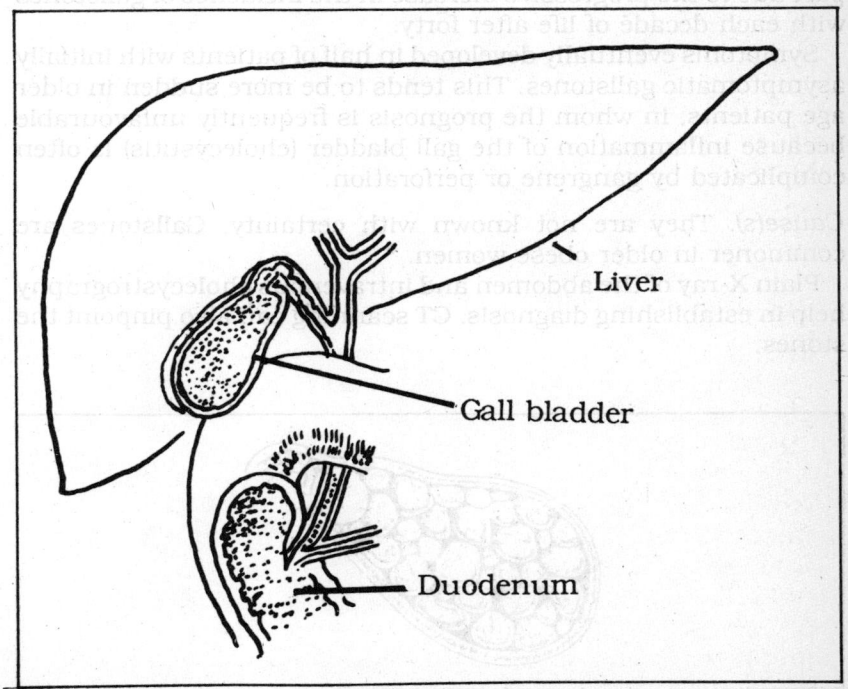

Gall bladder

The investigation of a jaundiced patient involves urine tests for bile and radiological examination for gallstones. Biochemical tests include an examination of the serum bilirubin which is raised in all forms of jaundice. The enzyme serum transaminase is raised when there is damage to the liver cells as in viral hepatitis. The enzyme serum alkaline phosphatase is raised in obstructive jaundice.

Liver biopsy is needed sometimes in doubtful cases.

Treatment. Obstructive jaundice is treated surgically. If there are gallstones, they can be removed. If the cause is cancerous growth, it can seldom be excised completely. When the obstruction cannot be overcome, the patient is likely to go downhill rapidly.

Gallstones

Gall bladder disease is one of the common conditions requiring abdominal operation in persons older than 60 years. This is in large part due to the progressive increase in the incidence of gallstones with each decade of life after forty.

Symptoms eventually developed in half of patients with initially asymptomatic gallstones. This tends to be more sudden in older age patients, in whom the prognosis is frequently unfavourable because inflammation of the gall bladder (cholecystitis) is often complicated by gangrene or perforation.

Cause(s). They are not known with certainty. Gallstones are commoner in older obese women.

Plain X-ray of the abdomen and intravenous cholecystrography help in establishing diagnosis. CT scanning can also pinpoint the stones.

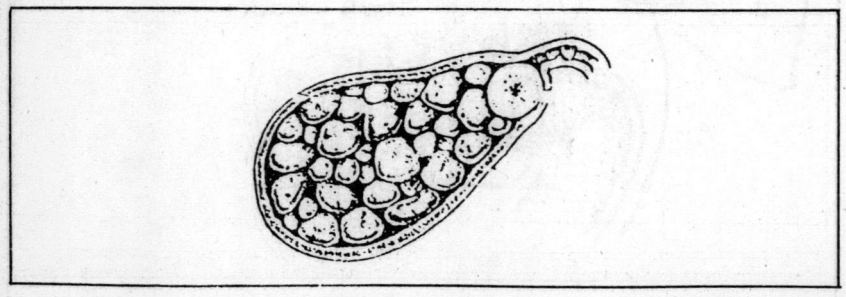

Gallstones

Treatment. There is no uniformity of opinion as to when or whether an elderly patient with 'silent' gallstones should be operated on; the decision depends largely on the relative risks of operation and the dangers of complications from the stones in a particular patient. The single large stone is more frequently associated with acute obstructive cholecystitis and its complications than are multiple small stones. Obesity and diabetes increase the risk. Advanced age in the absence of severe and debilitating disease does not contraindicate operation. Mortality is increased when emergency surgery is performed in the elderly.

Gall Bladder Infection (Cholecystitis)

It is more prevalent with advancing age and is more frequently accompanied by complications such as perforation.

Fever, abdominal findings and increase in the number of white blood cells (leukocytosis) are often less pronounced than expected. Jaundice is often seen because of the greater frequency of common bile duct stones.

Cause(s). Gall bladder stones make it more susceptible to infection.

Pain in the upper abdomen with fever, X-ray and CT scanning help in establishing diagnosis.

Treatment. Administration of appropriate antibiotics may help in abating infection and preventing complications. In case complications have already set in, urgent surgery is indicated to save the life of the patient.

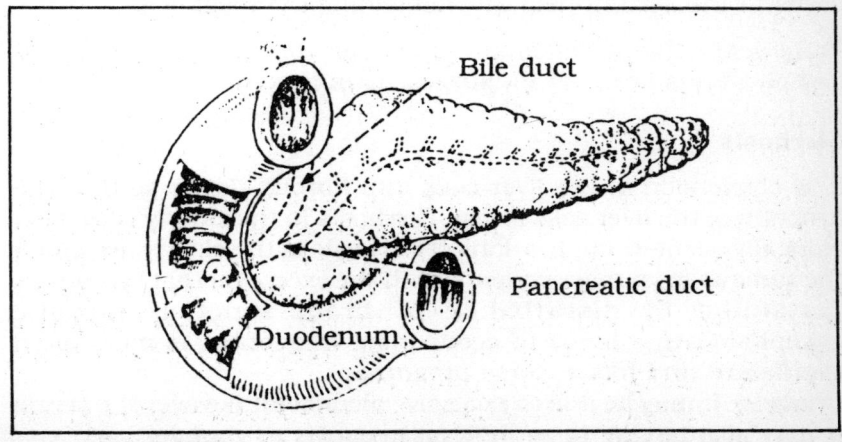

Pancreas

Acute Pancreatitis

Females are affected more often than males. Epigastric pain is the most common initial symptom. Fever, high pulse rate (tachycardia), and abdominal tenderness and guarding are characteristic, but may be less pronounced in the elderly.

Cause(s). They are many and varied.

Causes of Acute Pancreatitis in the Elderly
Biliary tract disease
Gallstones
Endocrine and metabolic diseases
Uraemia
Diabetes
Hypercalcemia
Medications
Thiazides
Furosemides
Cimetidine
Post-operative states
Post-endoscopy
Vascular (ischaemia)
Tumors (primary and metastatic).

History of the patient, physical examination, pancreatic enzyme levels in the serum, help in establishing the diagnosis.

Treatment. Giving of appropriate antibiotics may help. If complications have set in, surgery is indicated.

Cirrhosis

It is conversion of the liver cells into fibrous tissue so that the function of the liver cells is lost. Cirrhosis in the elderly is usually clinically silent. Complications of cirrhosis in the elderly are much the same as in younger patients, with the exception that symptoms pertaining to disturbance of brain function (hepatic encephalopathy) tends to occur more frequently, is more often overlooked and has a worse prognosis.

Cause(s). It may be due to excessive alcohol intake over the years. It may also be due to acute viral hepatitis in younger age.

History, physical examination, CT scan of the abdomen help in establishing the diagnosis.

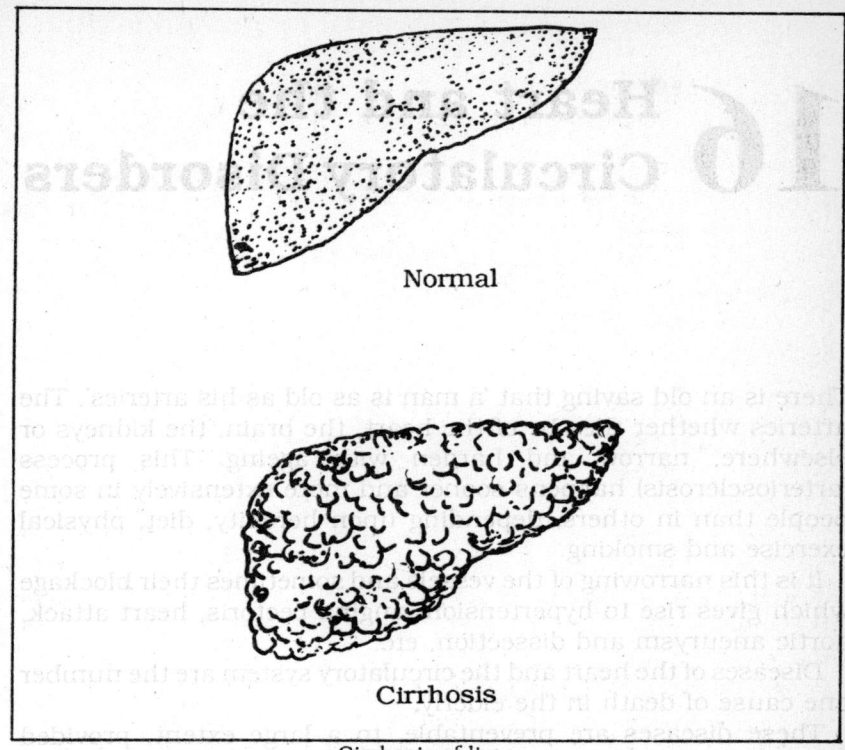

Normal

Cirrhosis

Cirrhosis of liver

Treatment. Development of repeated ascites or bleeding oesophageal varices are indications for surgery in the form of porto-systemic shunting procedure.

16 Heart and the Circulatory Disorders

There is an old saying that 'a man is as old as his arteries'. The arteries whether they be of the heart, the brain, the kidneys or elsewhere, narrow and harden with ageing. This process (arteriosclerosis) happens sooner and more extensively in some people than in others, depending upon heredity, diet, physical exercise and smoking.

It is this narrowing of the vessels and sometimes their blockage which gives rise to hypertension, angina pectoris, heart attack, aortic aneurysm and dissection, etc.

Diseases of the heart and the circulatory system are the number one cause of death in the elderly.

These diseases are preventable, to a large extent, provided adequate care is given to diet, physical exercise and avoidance of cigarette smoking. In America, these preventive measures have shown a declining trend of mortality and morbidity from these conditions.

Hypertension

There is no clear dividing line between the normal and the abnormal blood pressure. In elderly, normal is considered as upto 140/90 mm. Hypertension is any blood pressure above this level.

The prevalence of hypertension increases with age. Men are affected with hypertension more commonly before the age of 50; after menopause, however, women are affected more.

Cause(s). In 95 per cent of the cases, the cause is not known.

Specific cause can be identified in only approximately 5 per cent of the cases.

Specific Causes of Hypertension
Kidney disorders. Acromegaly (pituitary disorder). Adrenal cortex disorders (Cushing's disease). Hyperthyroidism. Hyperparathyroidism. Pheochromocytoma (tumour of the adrenal gland). Polycythemia (increased number of cells per units of blood). Oestrogen (female hormone) therapy.

Hypertension whether diastolic or systolic acts as a risk factor for cardiovascular disease. Myocardial infarction, sudden death due to coronary disease, angina pectoris and cerebrovascular accidents, are more common in hypertensives.

Treatment. Although there is conclusive evidence that normalization of blood pressure reduces the above hypertension-related complications, little information is currently available regarding the benefits of lowering the blood pressure in the elderly.

Methods other than drugs (non-pharmocologic) of reducing blood pressure have the advantage of not exposing the patient to any of the possible risks of drug therapy. Some of these methods such as reducing weight and restricting salt intake can be used in the elderly mild hypertensives.

The drug regimen should begin with lower doses than in younger patients. Increases should be made more gradually. Aggressive treatment with resultant hypotension in an older patient may be a greater short-term risk than the elevated blood pressure.

The usual first-line drug for managing hypertension in the elderly is a diuretic i.e., which causes increased production of urine. This single medication is often all that is needed to treat mild systolic and/or diastolic elevations. β-blocker (Atenolol) can be combined with the diuretic as the next step. A calcium channel blocker (Depin) can be added, if the desired effect is not produced with the above two.

Anti-hypertensive drugs are known to produce undesirable side-effects in most cases. If the side-effects are mild the patient may continue taking the drug; if they are severe, the patient may stop taking the drug. A knowledge of these side-effects is essential.

Anti-hypertensive Therapy in Elderly Patients

Step	Therapy
1	Diuretic
2	Diuretic + β blocker
3	Diuretic + β blocker + Calcium-channel blocker
4	All the above in adequate doses, plus any of the others such as captopril, hydralazine, methyldopa, clonidine, after assessing the contraindications.

Anti-hypertensive Drugs and their Side-effects

1. Diuretics (Hydrochlorothiazides)	Weakness, photo (light)-sensitivity, anaemia, impotence.
2. β-blockers	Bronchospasm, slow pulse, heart failure, confusion, depression, impotence.
3. Calcium-channel blockers	Oedema, heart failure, slow pulse.
4. Methyl-dopa, Clonidine	Dry mouth, gastro-intestinal dysfunction, sedation, impotence, gynaecomastia (swelling of the breasts), anaemia.
Hydralazine	Nasal congestion and watering from the eyes (lacrimation), fast pulse, blood and lung disorders.
Captopril	Skin rashes, fever, blood disorders.

An older hypertensive may also have angina or a history of myocardial infarction. In such a patient, excessive or rapid lowering of blood pressure may be risky. Diuretics, β-blockers and calcium-channel blockers are especially useful for him in low dosages.

When kidney is not functioning properly, doses of the drugs, particularly atenolol, captopril which are excreted by the kidney, need to be reduced.

In a diabetic hypertensive, particular attention should be paid to maintaining total body potassium levels at as near normal as possible. Over-aggressive correction of potassium loss should be avoided in those diabetics with kidney function insufficiency.

Angina Pectoris

The symptoms of angina in an elderly may differ somewhat from those in a younger person. Although chest pain is often a presenting finding, its presence or absence is not diagnostic. Angina may present with symptoms as diverse as breathlessness (dyspnoea), lethargy, wheezing and/or mental confusion.

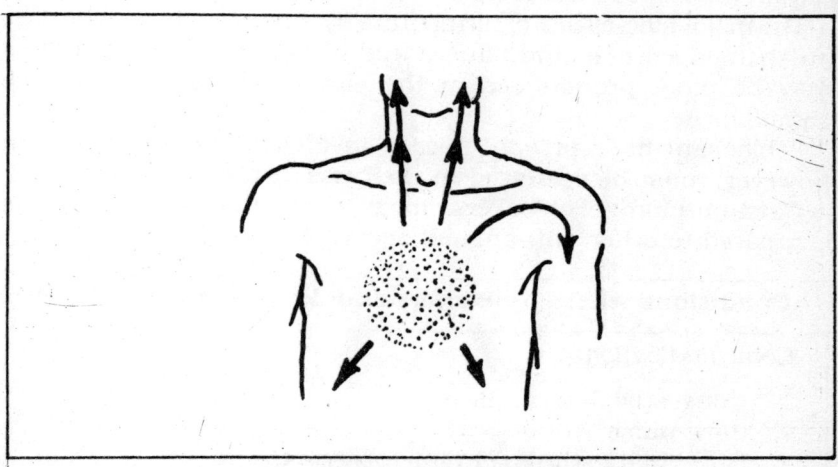

Anginal pain and its radiation

If an older person's activities are limited by arthritis, respiratory or other problems, he may not be able to physically exert

Risk Factors for Angina Pectoris
Obesity
Hypertension
Cigarette smoking
Emotional and/or physical stress
Hyperthyroidism
Anaemia

sufficiently to be aware of the anginal symptoms. Diminished awareness of pain or the existence of gastro-intestinal or musculo-skeletal chest pain may similarly obscure the diagnosis.

Cause(s). Atherosclerosis in the coronary arteries and their subsequent narrowing is the main cause.

Treatment. A search for treatable risk or contributing factors such as hypertension, hyperthyroidism, or anaemia should be made and remedied as far as possible.

The main line of treatment for angina pectoris includes medication such as the nitrates, β-blockers, and the newer calcium-channel blockers. They act by reducing myocardial oxygen requirement and increasing coronary artery blood flow.

The major side-effects of nitrates are hypotension, headache, fast pulse (tachycardia), and nausea and vomiting. These symptoms may be more pronounced in the elderly and so may reduce compliance.

β-blockers have proven efficacy in angina pectoris. Caution however, must be exercised in their use in the elderly.

Calcium-channel blockers have relatively few side-effects compared to other anti-anginal agents.

Conditions where β-blockers should be used with Care

Contraindications

1. Congestive heart failure
2. Slow pulse
3. Bronchial asthma/chronic obstructive airway disease
4. Diabetes mellitus
5. Hypotension

Side-effects

1. Bronchospasm
2. Hypotension
3. Congestive heart failure
4. Slow pulse
5. Raynaud's phenomenon (blanching of hands and feet when exposed to cold)
6. Central nervous system (CNS) disturbances, depression, hallucinations
7. Impotence
8. Hypoglycemia (low blood sugar)

The goal of drug therapy for angina is to maintain a functionally independent life style free of signs and symptoms. Therapy should start with nitrates and progress to, β-blockers. There is good evidence that the two agents may have an additive effect in the control of symptoms.

Care must be taken to choose an appropriate calcium-channel blocker as a third agent. Diltiazem may be safely used with both nitrates and β-blockers.

In the past decade, there has been widespread application of coronary artery by-pass surgery. More recently, percutaneous transluminal coronary angioplasty i.e., dilation of the narrowed arteries by passing a ballooned catheter in them, has been tried in the treatment of refractory angina pectoris. Despite the modest increase in risk with advancing age, both coronary by-pass surgery and transluminal angioplasty represent attractive therapeutic approaches for the elde.·ly patient with medically refractory angina pectoris.

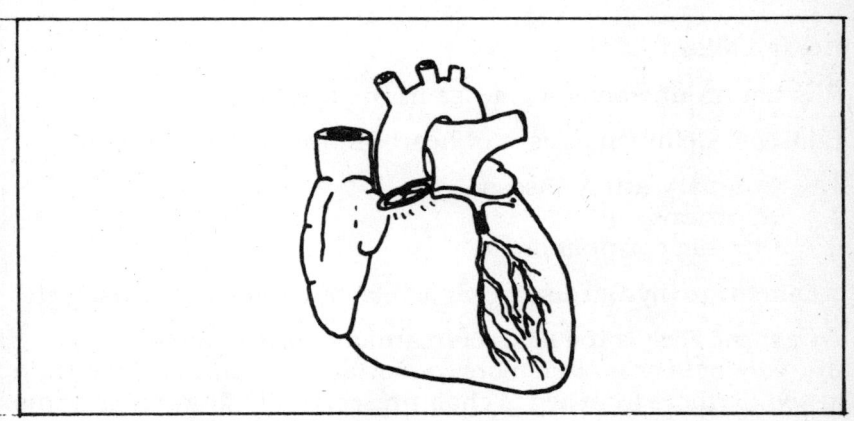

Coronary artery blockage

Acute Myocardial Infarction (Heart Attack)

Acute myocardial infarction (MI) continues to present a diagnostic and therapeutic problem in old age. In an often-quoted study of 597 chronically institutionalised patients aged 65 and older, with acute MI, only 19 per cent presented with classic chest pain symptoms. Sudden dyspnoea or exacerbation of previously controlled heart failure was the most common presenting complaint (20%). Acute confusion (12%), sudden death (7%) syncope (7%), hemiplegia (6%), peripheral arterial occlusion (5%), vertigo (5%) and palpitations (4%), were other common presentations. The high prevalence of dyspnoea in the elderly compared with younger populations with acute MI, may relate to the superimposition of infarction on an already damaged heart by virtue of age, resulting in collection of blood in the lung vessels.

The mortality from acute MI rises dramatically with age, averaging 40 per cent in those older than 70 years, a rate at least twice that of younger individuals. The elderly are also much more likely to present with heart failure, pulmonary oedema or cardiogenic shock.

Cause(s). Narrowing (atherosclerosis) of the coronary arteries and their blockage.

Treatment. If the patient is not in pain but restless only, diazepam (Valium) or chlorpromazine (Largactil) may be appropriate.

Besides that oxygen and diuretics are indicated.

Early mobilization is the best defence against thrombophlebitis and pulmonary embolism.

Heart Failure

It is not an uncommon disease in the elderly.

Cause(s). Common causes of heart failure in the elderly are:

1.   Coronary artery disease.
2.   Hypertension.
3.   Chronic cor-pulmonale.

Others are thyroid disease, anaemia, pulmonary embolism, etc.

Treatment. Rest is the basis of treatment for the failing heart, but the older patient is often more comfortable resting in a chair than in bed. To move from bed to chair preserves mobility and prevents stiffening of the joints. For the same reason it is desirable to allow the patient to walk to the lavatory as soon as he can do so. If kept in bed, the patient will be more comfortable when he is well propped up with plenty of pillows.

Sleep is essential but does not come easily to the patient who is breathless (dyspnoeic).

An injection of morphine is helpful. Other sedative drugs including diazepam (Valium) and chlorpromazine (Largactil) may also be helpful.

Oxygen is indicated in a cyanosed and breathless patient. The patient is likely to have a poor appetite because he is breathless and because he has congestion of the stomach and liver. Salt may be restricted but fluids can be given freely.

When the heart fails, the blood flow to the kidneys is reduced. This leads to retention of sodium in the body and the consequent oedema. Diuretics encourage excretion of sodium and water through the kidney. They are the most important drugs in the treatment of heart failure. The disappearance of the retained fluid is most easily demonstrated by the patient's improved condition and rapid loss of weight. The best way to assess their effect is to weigh the patient regularly.

Some diuretics act quickly, others more slowly. The most useful quick-acting diuretics are frusemide (Lasix) and bumetanide (Bumet). Given in the morning, the patient passes urine during the day and sleeps well at night. If these diuretics do not suit the patient, the longer-acting preparations can be used. Most diuretics cause loss of potassium in the urine and this must be replaced. Potassium chloride can be given as a tablet or as an effervescent drink. Old people sometimes dislike potassium supplements as they often cause minor degrees of indigestion.

A most valuable drug, especially when the patient's heart failure is associated with atrial fibrillation, is digoxin (Lanoxin). It slows the pulse, strengthens the heart beat and controls atrial fibrillation if this is present. The older patient needs small doses. Digoxin toxicity is common, especially in patients depleted of potassium by diuretics. Digoxin toxicity is manifested by disturbance of heart rhythm, confusion, diarrhoea, nausea and vomiting.

Infective Endocarditis

It is inflammation of the inner lining of the heart including the valves inside it. Formerly seen in younger people, it is being seen now in older people, more often males above 60.

The following atypical presentations are common in older people and frequently lead to a delay in diagnosis:

1. Fever and murmur are often absent.
2. Neurological symptoms and signs are common, their presence increases the mortality rate to 75 per cent.
3. Urinary symptoms occur frequently.
4. Congestive heart failure (53%) and uraemia (44%) often occur.
5. Skin lesions (bleeding spots) occur in 33 per cent of cases.
6. Psychiatric symptoms (depression, confusion) are common and may be the only presenting signs.

Cause(s). Although underlying rheumatic heart disease still represents an important predisposing condition in old age, different valvular disorders such as calcific aortic stenosis, mitral valve prolapse, mitral annular calcification, and prosthetic valves, represent increasingly common foci for endocarditis in the elderly.

Surgical procedures such as dental extraction, drainage of an abscess, urinary or pelvic infection or operation, insertion of a pacemaker, which may lead to entry of bacteria into the blood stream, carry a risk of causing infective endocarditis. The risk is even greater when intravenous drugs are given in the hospital surroundings.

Common microorganisms associated with infective endocarditis include:

1. Streptococcus viridens, most commonly seen in elderly persons following dental procedures.
2. Staphylococcus aureus associated with surgical procedures, particularly heart valve replacement.
3. Gram negative organisms associated with gastrointestinal tract manipulation.
4. Fungus associated with immunologic deficiencies and surgical valve replacement.

Diagnosis is often overlooked in old age because of: (1) the failure to even consider endocarditis in the elderly, (2) the absence of typical features.

Blood cultures for different microorganisms help in establishing the diagnosis. Other features that help in the diagnosis are: anaemia, presence of red blood cells in the urine (hematuria), abnormal kidney functions, elevated ESR.

Treatment. It is based on the results of the blood cultures and the sensitivity of the isolated organisms to particular drugs.

The treatment of choice for enterococcal endocarditis is penicillin G or ampicillin combined with aminoglycoside (i.e., gentamicin).

Pencillin-sensitive streptococci (S. viridens and S. bovis) are effectively treated with high doses of penicillin. Staphylococcal endocarditis is treated with penicillinase-resistant penicillin often combined with aminoglycosides or rifampicin.

A poorer prognosis occurs in the elderly because of common delays in diagnosis, more frequent infection with S. aureus, and a higher incidence of underlying cardiovascular disease. Mortality rates reach 40 to 60 per cent.

Irregular Pulse (Arrhythmia)

Irregular pulse due to various defects in conductance of electrical impulse in the heart, is a common problem in the older people. These irregularities are of various types depending upon the site and type of the conduction defect.

Symptoms associated with arrhythmias may range from a mild 'light-headed' feeling with occasional palpitations, momentary unconsciousness (syncope) and sudden death. In every case, careful evaluation and timely intervention are potentially life-saving. The presence of a ventricular rhythm disturbance in the elderly is often associated with an increased risk of sudden death. Although many elderly have occasional premature ventricular contractions (PVC), the presence of symptoms, previously existing structural heart disease and the frequency of PVC influences the ultimate prognosis.

Classification of Arrhythmias Commonly Seen in the Elderly

Fast irregular (Tachy-arrhythmia)

Sinus tachycardia
Paroxysmal supraventricular tachycardia
Atrial flutter
Ventricular tachycardia

Slow irregular (Bradycardia)

Sinus bradycardia
Sinus node impairment
Complete heart block

Cause(s). Arrhythmias are caused by defects in the conduction system of the heart, due to damage by atherosclerosis.

Treatment. Careful evaluation and treatment with an appropriate anti-arrhythmic drug is indicated to decrease the risk of sudden death.

When the irregularity is not adequately responsive to drugs and endangers the life of the patient, an artificial pacemaker for the heart is implanted. This pacemaker now sets the electrical impulse in the heart and regulates the heart-beat of the patient.

A pacemaker is usually needed in the older patients whose hearts have borne many injuries during the process of ageing. Complete heart block and sick sinus syndrome need the pacemaker most often.

A pacemaker may be needed temporarily to tide over an emergency, or on a permanent basis. The patient and his relations are made aware of the small but significant pacemaker-induced complications. Abrupt loss of pacing due to battery failure, fibrosis around the catheter site, myocardial perforation, wire fracture, or electrode dislodgment, may result in marked bradycardia or the stoppage of the heart.

Aortic Aneurysms

Wall of the aorta can dilate due to weakness in its structure. This dilation is called aneurysm. Aortic aneurysms are common in the elderly. They increase in severity in the same patient with increasing age.

Cause(s). They are caused usually by atherosclerosis occuring in in the larger vessels, in this case the aorta. They may occur in the thoracic part of the aorta or the abdominal.

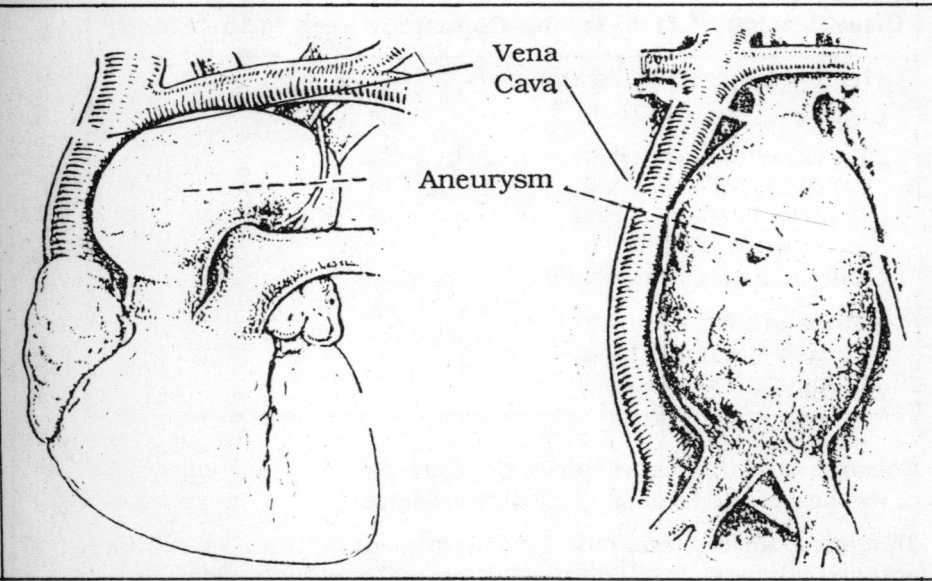

Aneurysm thoracic aorta   Aneurysm abdominal aorta

Diagnosis is usually made on routine physical examination and may be confirmed by X-rays; the majority of the aneurysms contain calcium deposits, making the lesion radiopaque. Ultrasonography can also help in diagnosis.

Treatment. Aneurysms larger than 6 cms. in size are usually considered for surgery, but the surgical mortality is substantially high.

Aneurysms can rupture and cause instantaneous death. Some patients with known aneurysms, however, do survive for years.

Patients with aortic aneurysms are known to simultaneously suffer from angina pectoris, myocardial infarction and heart failure which need to be cared for simultaneously.

Aortic Dissection

It is a length-wise rupture within the wall of the aorta whereby the blood flows in the lumen of the aorta as well as in the lumen created by the rupture. If the rupture opens on the outside of the wall of the aorta, all the blood will flow out into the thorax or abdomen and cause sudden death.

Aortic dissection is a medical emergency that most commonly occurs in men over fifty years of age. It is characterized by the sudden onset of excruciating chest pain radiating to the scapula in the back; the pain, however, may also be felt in the neck, jaw, arm, abdomen and/or the leg.

There are two major sites of aortic dissection: the ascending aorta, representing approximately 70 per cent of the cases and the descending aorta occuring in approximately 30 per cent of the cases.

The condition has to be differentiated from many other emergencies that can occur in the chest or the abdomen.

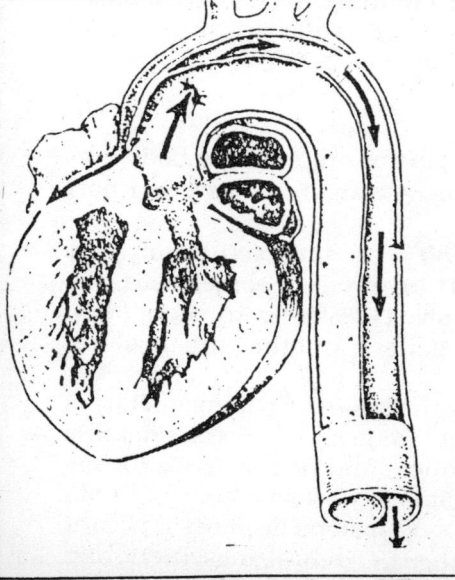

Dissecting aneurysm thoracic aorta

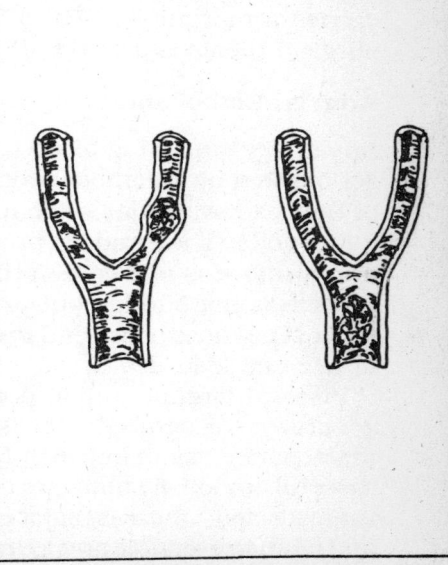

Embolus blocking an artery

Differential Diagnosis of Aortic Dissection
Acute myocardial infarction (heart attack) Pericarditis (inflammation of the covering of the heart) Pulmonary embolus Pneumothorax (air in the pleura) Biliary colic Acute cholecystitis Appendicitis

Cause(s). In a majority of the cases, the cause is atherosclerosis in the aorta.

Contrast arteriography helps in making an accurate diagnosis. The computed tomography (CT) scan with contrast, of the aorta can pinpoint the site of the aortic dissection.

Treatment. Rapid diagnosis and treatment is essential, as mortality is very high in an untreated case. The initial treatment is largely medical. The blood pressure which is usually high, must be lowered with anti-hypertensive medication.

Mortality is higher in cases of the ascending aorta dissection. Surgical repair of the lesion is called for even though the operation carries a high risk of death. Medical management in such cases carries a mortality of 70 to 80 per cent, while death risk from surgical repair is around 40 per cent.

Arterial Embolism

Any artery supplying blood to any part or organ of the body may get blocked by an embolus or a plug, arising from any other part of the cardiovascular system.

More often it is a sudden process (80%) causing excruciating pain and numbness and cold in the part involved. In some cases, the process is not sudden but progressive (12%) or even silent (8%). Half of the these cases end up with gangrene of the limb involved, or even sudden death.

Visceral (organ) emboli occur with greater frequency than is generally recognized. It is well known that considerable discrepancy exists between the clinical and necropsy diagnosis. Visceral emboli, if small, are often clinically over-looked or remain unsuspected, whereas major embolic occlusions display significant and often irreversible and lethal changes. Cerebral, mesenteric and renal emboli are not uncommon, and they are often the cause of serious complications or death.

Cause(s). The embolus causing the obstruction to the blood supply may arise from: (1) the thrombus on the inside wall of the heart involved in myocardial infarction, (2) thrombus arising from the left atrium of the heart in cases of atrial fibrillation and (3) a dislodged plaque of the arteriosclerotic process in a large blood vessel such as the aorta.

Diagnosis is often made from (1) the history of the loss of blood supply to the part, and (2) the underlying heart disease.

Treatment. As a first step, the patient should be placed in the head-up position with the involved limb protected from pressure.

Heparin should be administered intravenously as soon as possible.

Embolectomy (removal of the embolus) is the method of choice for managing arterial emboli.

Drug treatment with vasodilater substances such as nicotinic acid is likely to be tried but is not often of much help. More important is intensive treatment with antibiotics if there is suggestion of infection around the toes.

Elevation of the limb and application of local heat are the two most ill-advised procedures that should be scrupulously avoided.

Venous Thrombosis

This is the blockage of the veins with clotted blood. When the clot dislodges from its site of origin, it may go and settle in the lung (pulmonary) veins and block them.

Cause(s). The increased frequency of vein thrombosis of the leg seems to be directly correlated with a progressive enlargement of the calf veins, which occurs with advancing years.

It is also frequently seen as a post-operative complication, or in patients bed-ridden as a result of a chronic disease.

Treatment. It depends on the location and extent of thrombosis. Involvement of the saphenous veins in the lower limbs, or of the upper limbs rarely, if ever, requires bed rest and elevation. In the absence of spreading thrombosis, and lack of oedema or pain, application of an ice-bandage and use of an anti-inflammatory agent may overcome the local process within a few days to 2 weeks.

In older patients, it is often desirable to use anti-coagulant drugs as a prophylaxis to venous thromboembolism, in those undergoing surgical procedures. Once anticoagulant treatment is established, the patient should be encouraged to move his leg and to walk as much as possible, but he should not sit in a chair for long periods as this will increase the swelling of his leg. A crape bandage helps to control the swelling and an elastic stocking will be useful afterwards.

Pulmonary Embolism

The classic symptoms include pleuritic chest pain, sweating and spitting of blood (haemoptysis). Breathlessness occurs in cases of massive embolism. It is a frequent cause of death in the elderly.

Cause(s). Most pulmonary emboli originate in the deep veins of the pelvis and lower extremities, with venous stasis a causative factor. There is often no prior history of leg pain or swelling.

Predisposing Factors
1. Prolonged immobilization (bed rest)   2. Varicose veins   3. Cancer   4. Oestrogen therapy (female hormone)   5. Pelvic surgery   6. Congestive heart failure

The classic symptoms of sudden onset of pleuritic chest pain, dyspnoea and haemoptysis may be confused with other disorders in the older patient, or be missed completely. When these symptoms occur in the presence of a normal chest X-ray, there should be a high degree of suspicion.

Treatment. The best way to reduce death and disability from pulmonary embolism is to prevent the formation of thrombi in the venous system of the lower extremities.

A case of massive pulmonary embolism with collapse will need treatment for shock. If his heart is still beating, the foot of the bed should be raised and oxygen given by a mask.

An immediate intravenous injection of heparin is given while a decision is made about further treatment. It may be decided to try and dissolve the embolus with the fibrinolyic drug, streptokinase (streptase). This is given by infusion after an initial slow intravenous injection.

Pulmonary embolism and cardiac infarction are the two causes of death in the older patient. They raise the question of resuscitation. Cardiac massage is necessary and helpful in some cases.

17 Respiratory Disorders

Ageing causes many changes in the respiratory system. The ribs and the chest wall expand less with inspiration. There is some bending forward of the thorax at the spinal column which allows less expansion of the lungs. The lungs become less elastic and in some places, walls between the alveoli break and disappear. All this results in diminished capacity of gas exchange in the lungs, so that a little exertion makes an older person breathe at a higher rate per minute, and he feels breathless.

The secretions of the lungs also show a diminished capacity to defend the inner lining of the airways and the alveoli against bacteria. The older persons thus are more susceptible to lung infections such as pneumonia. Excessive alcohol intake further reduces the power of the lungs against infecting bacteria or viruses.

The greatest harm to the respiratory system occurs from cigarette smoking. Smoking extending over decades causes chronic bronchitis, emphysema and lung cancer.

Quitting cigarettes even after many years of smoking, can make an older person feel healthier and less liable to diseases that the smoking causes.

Pneumonia

It is inflammation of the lung or part of it. Pneumonia is a common disease of the older people, and is liable to cause death.

General immune response (bodily resistance) in older people is feeble and the local defence mechanisms of the lungs are also not very effective. The result is a more frequent occurence of pneumonia with increased severity.

Pneumonia may be the primary disease occurring in a healthy lung, or a secondary process in an already diseased lung having chronic bronchitis, bronchiectasis or even cancer.

In primary pneumonia, the bacteria may be aspirated from the mouth cavity or upper respiratory tract. In a secondary process, the bacteria may spread in contiguous parts of the lungs from a focus of infection already present in the lungs.

As pneumonia develops, the alveoli of the lungs get filled with an exudate due to the infection. The exudate replaces the air in the lung and the affected parts are said to become consolidated. A consolidated lung cannot take up oxygen. If the pneumonia is extensive, it interferes with breathing and may lead to cyanosis (bluish tinge) and hypoxia (less of oxygen in the blood). Toxaemia from the infection adds to the patient's illness.

The clinical picture of pneumonia in the elderly is quite variable. Usual symptoms including chills, sweats, chest pain, and sputum production may be present, but one should not rely on these for mak `ng a diagnosis. Subtle changes in mental status, exacerbation of underlying chronic illness such as congestive heart failure may be the only expressed features.

The pulse rate is usually high. The most constant feature is an increase in the rate of respiration. Some cyanosis is common. The patient looks pinched, but his nostrils are dilated. He may be too weak to raise sputum; if he can, it is likely to be purulent.

Often the symptoms are not those of chest disease at all, but of cerebral hypoxia (lack of oxygen in the brain); the patient becoming confused, restless and noisy.

Complications of pneumonia are also more common in the elderly. These are bacteremia (bacteria in the blood), empyema (pus in the pleura) and meningitis (inflammation of meninges), all leading to increased mortality. The reason for this appears to be the age-related decline in immunologic defence mechanisms.

Cause(s). Primary bacterial pneumonia is usually caused by Streptococcus pneumonia, and the secondary by Streptococcus haemolyticus, Staphylococcus aureus, other gram negative organisms or even anaerobic bacteria (those which need no oxygen to grow). The bacteria causing secondary pneumonia are more destructive to the lungs.

Suspecting pneumonia from the variable clinical features, in particular, high pulse rate and high respiration rate, is the most important step towards diagnosis. X-ray of the chest establishes the diagnosis. Sputum examination very often helps in finding out the causative organisms.

Treatment. Giving an antibiotic to eradicate the infection is the first essential. To determine the most suitable antibiotic, it is necessary to obtain a specimen of sputum for bacterological examination. Before the infecting organism is identified, treatment is started immediately with a broad-spectrum antibiotic, which works well in most cases. Where oral treatment is not possible, the drugs may be given intramuscularly or intraveneously.

Pneumonia, especially in a patient already suffering from bronchitis and emphysema, may well provoke respiratory failure and oxygen must be given. Most of the restlessness of the elderly patient of pneumonia, is due to hypoxia.

The older patient with pneumonia is especially liable to dehydration i.e., less of water in the body. Not only is this bad in itself, but it may lead to the complication of renal failure, which adds to the gravity of the disease. To prevent dehydration, special attention must be paid to patient's fluid intake, and this is much the most important aspect of his diet. If he is not eating, he will need at least two litres of fluid per day. This can be given by mouth. With very ill patients, it is often easier, to give fluids by intra-gastric drip.

The patient should be made to sit up, as this makes breathing easier. He should be allowed out of bed for short periods as soon as there is any sign of improvement.

Chronic Bronchitis

It is defined clinically by the presence of a productive cough on most days at least 3 months of the year for more than two consecutive years, in the absence of any other specific disease like tuberculosis or bronchiectasis.

Cause(s). The cause most often is tobacco smoking. The mucous membrane lining the bronchial tree, the finely branching air passages connecting the trachea to the alveoli of the lung, is sensitive to tobacco smoke and other irritants. It responds by becoming swollen and secreting more mucus. The patient then develops a smoker's cough with mucoid sputum. To this may be added the effect of infection when the sputum becomes purulent, and the cough more severe. The extra secretions in the bronchi impede the flow of air in and out of the lungs and the patient becomes breathless. In addition, there may be spasm of the bronchi, further narrowing their lumen. This increases the airways' obstruction and the patient develops a wheeze. All these changes are at first reversible but repeated infection and continued exposure to tobacco permanently damage the bronchi and lungs, causing increasing disability.

Cigarette smoking is the major cause of the disease. Heredity, air pollution, occupation, and childhood respiratory infections may increase the damage done by cigarette smoking, but seldom cause the disease by themselves.

The history of tobacco-smoking and presence of cough and breathlessness points towards chronic bronchitis; X-ray of the chest and lung function tests can clinch the diagnosis.

Treatment. Chronic bronchitis needs help when an acute exacrebation occurs due to a superadded infection. The patient needs an antibiotic. The infection is caused primarily by Hemophilus influenzae and Streptococcus pneumoniae but many other organisms are involved secondarily. The antibiotic usually preferred is amoxycillin. This is given in high dosage at first in an effort to eradicate the hemophilus from the sputum. After the first week, lower doses can be used or a change can be made to co-trimoxazole (Septran), or caphalexin (Ceporex). Antibiotics are continued as long as the sputum is purulent.

The patient with bronchitis has copious sputum, and assisted coughing supervised by the physiotherapist plays an important role in treatment, clearing the air passages and helping him to breathe. Steam inhalations loosen the sputum and make it easier for the patient to cough effectively.

The patient also needs an antispasmodic to relieve his wheezing. The best is salbutamol (Ventolin), or terbutaline (Bricanyl). These have fewer side-effects on the heart, brain and bladder than ephedrine and isoprenaline which were previously employed. They can be given by mouth, injection or inhalation.

The patient must quit smoking.

Emphysema

Emphysema is defined as a condition of the lungs characterized by increased beyond the normal in the size of the alveoli with destructive changes in their walls.

Cause(s). Smoking cigarettes can cause emphysema as well as chronic bronchitis. A patient of emphysema is usually a smoker of many years' standing having breathlessness on exertion. He may be having cough and phlegm also. His chest is expanded, and lungs full of air, so that he can take little of outside air in his lungs with each breath and has difficulty in breathing out air.

Diagnosis is made from the history of the patient as being a smoker and having exertional breathlessness. X-ray of the chest shows the expanded lungs, and the lung function tests indicate the diagnosis.

Treatment. The first step to treatment is stoppage of smoking. This leads to decreased phlegm and some improvement in breathing.

If there is infection in the lungs with purulent phlegm, antibiotics will be needed to check and remove the infection.

If patient is severely breathless and cyanosed, oxygen administration is essential.

If the patient has developed chronic obstructive airway disease, which many of them do, and has heart failure as well, then diuretics are needed to bring the patient out of the heart failure. Continuous oxygen therapy has prolonged life in these patients.

Asthma

It usually starts in younger patients. Older patients having asthma have continuation of the disease acquired at a younger age.

The patient has attacks of breathlessness and wheeze. While younger patients have periods when there is no breathlessness, in older patients freedom from breathlessness is hardly there.

Cause(s) The older patient may have history of allergy in the family and he may be allergic to house dust, moulds or fungi or even pollens.

Fairly often, it is the chronic infection in the lungs, which gives rise to symptoms of asthma.

The diagnosis is established from the history of the patient, physical examination, X-ray of the chest, lung function tests and the allergy testing, all combined together.

Treatment. The patient may be treated symptomatically, i.e., by removal of his bronchospasm by drugs, oxygen and intravenous fluids, as well as antibiotics, if needed.

The patient can be given immunotherapy injections if he has been found to be allergic to certain outside substances in his environments.

Many a time, existence of asthma for many years, even decades, leads to structural changes in the lungs, which are difficult to cure.

Tuberculosis

While a younger patient with tuberculosis presents with fever, night sweats, weight loss and anorexia, such a presentation may not occur in the elderly. Cough may be present, but there may be no fever. General weakness, diminished appetite and loss of weight may be the only symptoms.

Cause(s). Lung tuberculosis is caused by inhalation of tubercle bacilli excreted through the lung secretions of another patient.

In an elderly person, alcoholism, malnutrition, diabetes, cancer, renal dialysis, and treatment with immunoppressive drugs, are known to reactivate old tuberculosis lesions acquired in the earlier life.

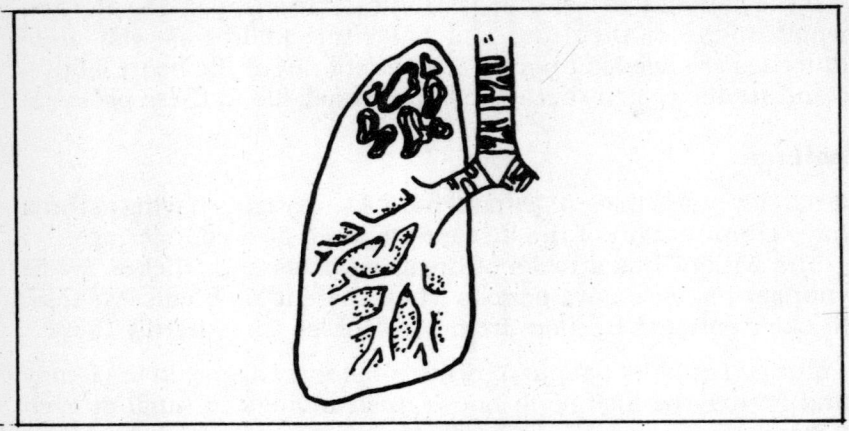

Tuberculous lung

History of the patient, coupled with X-ray of the chest and sputum examination for tubercle bacilli, establish the diagnosis.

Treatment. It is on the same lines as in younger patients. In case of renal or liver derangement of function, the dosage of the drugs is reduced as a excretion of the anti-tuberculosis drugs may be hindered. Duration of administration depends upon the response.

Lung Cancer

Cancer of the lung is fast increasing in incidence in older patients.

The patient may have no symptoms at all, if the cancer is localized and very small. If it is larger, the patient may have cough, phlegm, blood in the phlegm (haemoptysis), breathlessness. He may be weak, emaciated, with loss of appetite and weight. All this depends upon the size and site of the disease.

Cause(s). Smoking cigarettes over many years and decades is the only cause in the vast majority of the cases.

Diagnosis is established through history, physical examination, X-ray of the chest. Bronchoscopy wherein the lesion may be directly seen and its biopsy taken, establishes the diagnosis.

Treatment. Resection of the involved lung is still the primary

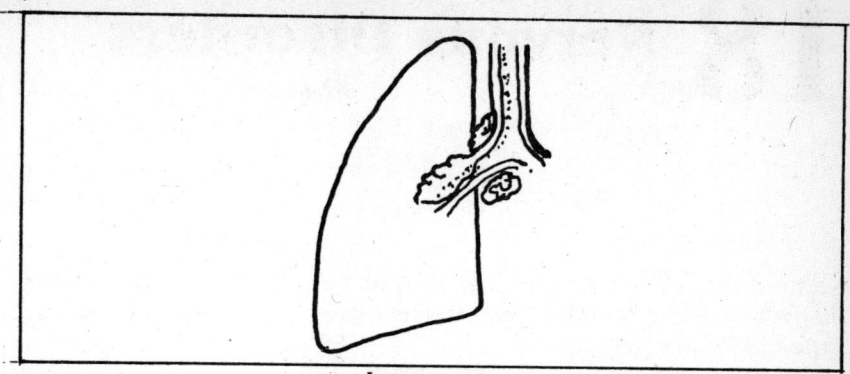

Lung cancer

therapy in squamous cancer of the lung. Five-year survival rates approaching 69 per cent are reported with tumours less than 3 cm diameter in size and without spread in other parts of the body (metastasis). Radiation therapy is used as an adjunct to surgery and for removal of symptoms (palliation).

Chemotherapy (use of anti-cancer drugs) in small-cell or oat-cell carcinoma with multiple drugs and as adjunct with radiation, is known to cause remission in a large percentage of patients. But metastasis to the brain and other sites in the lung occur early with this carcinoma.

18 Nervous Disorders

Some diseases of the nervous system in older people are due to disorders of the blood supply to the brain; these include various types of brain strokes.

There are others in which the brain cells are involved. In these there may be structural defects in the cells, as happens in cases of dementias of various types. Diminution in the number of brain cells occurs with ageing and this diminution in certain parts causes specific deficiencies in function. Some disorders of the brain cells have no microscopic change in them, yet there are biochemical changes which result in certain diseases, as for example parkinsonism.

In many other brain disorders, the brain as a whole does not function well. These include depression, anxiety, neurosis, hypochondriasis, etc.

While we know, to an extent, how the brain controls movements, sensations and regulation of the body, we do not know enough about the collective work of the brain, i.e., the mind.

Older people, many a time, suffer from all the above disorders at one time, i.e., disorders of blood supply, anatomical defects of the cells and also the malfunctioning mind.

Unfortunately, we can hardly do much for these disorders, and day-to-day care of the patient is all that we can do or hope for.

Brain Stroke

The arteries which supply the brain are subject to narrowing (arteriosclerosis) in the same way as are the coronary arteries, the aorta and the other vessels. A narrowed artery in the brain may be blocked by a plug of detached atheroma (thrombus), thus cutting off all blood supply to that part of the brain. A hardened blood vessel may as well rupture, denying blood to the part which it normally supplies. Brain cells suffer instantly, should the circulation become inadequate or cut.

Stoppage of blood supply to a part of a brain may be transient or permanent, less severe or more severe. The symptoms produced as a result of it, vary accordingly.

A patient may experience transient attacks of weakness (hemiperesis) or loss of sensation (hemianaesthesia) of one side of the body. These transient attacks are often due to atheromatous occlusion of the main neck arteries, or due to platelet, cholesterol or fibrin emboli that arise in these vessels and are carried to the cerebral arteries.

A major stroke is one in which considerable neurologic deficit occurs and remains even after a few weeks. The clinical picture differs very little from that seen at other ages, but it is more difficult for a very old person to survive a massive cerebral infarction, or if he does so, to achieve an excellent recovery of function. Mental disturbances with forgetfulness, loss of interest, inability to persevere, blunting of determination, and failure to understand, are the chief bars to successful rehabilitation. All depend on how much of the former youthful vigorous personality remains at the time of the stroke in old age and how strong the wish is to remain alive and independent.

Cause(s). Atherosclerosis (narrowing and hardening) of the vessels, supplying blood to the brain, is the main cause.

CT scan can help identify an acute brain infarction (due to cutting of blood supply) within 24 to 48 hours, and a haemorrhage (bleeding) immediately.

Examination of the cerebrospinal fluid (CSF) is indicated in cases in which subarachnoid haemorrhage is suspected in the absence of focal neurological signs.

Treatment. It has two aspects: the original emergency and the subsequent rehabilitation.

In the immediate treatment of a major stroke affecting an elderly patient, nursing care is more important than any specific medical therapy. The main principles are maintenance of a free airway and adequate hydration and nutrition. Preservation of a good systemic circulation combined with prevention of respiratory and urinary infection are other important points. Pressure sores have to be prevented.

Dentures, if there, should be removed and the patient nursed in the semi-prone position. He can be kept on his side by a pillow at his back. The semi-prone position keeps the tongue forward and maintains the patient's airways. The foot of the bed may be raised to facilitate drainage of secretions from the mouth. Regular suction may be needed to clear the pharynx, and if there are signs of oxygen lack, the patient should be given oxygen by a nasal catheter.

If the patient is in coma, he should be given fluids by intravenous catheter. If he is not deeply unconscious and has a cough reflex, fluids may be given by gastric drip. He will inevitably be incontinent and should have an indwelling catherter with closed drainage for passing urine. Such a patient runs a great risk of developing pressure sores and should receive two-hourly turning.

Patients with cerebral embolism are treated with anticoagulants. Antibiotics may be needed for a chest or urinary infection.

In the elderly, risk factors must be carefully weighed against possible benefits and expected life-span at the time of surgery. Emergency surgery may be required for removal of blood clots in the posterior part that show evidence of expansion.

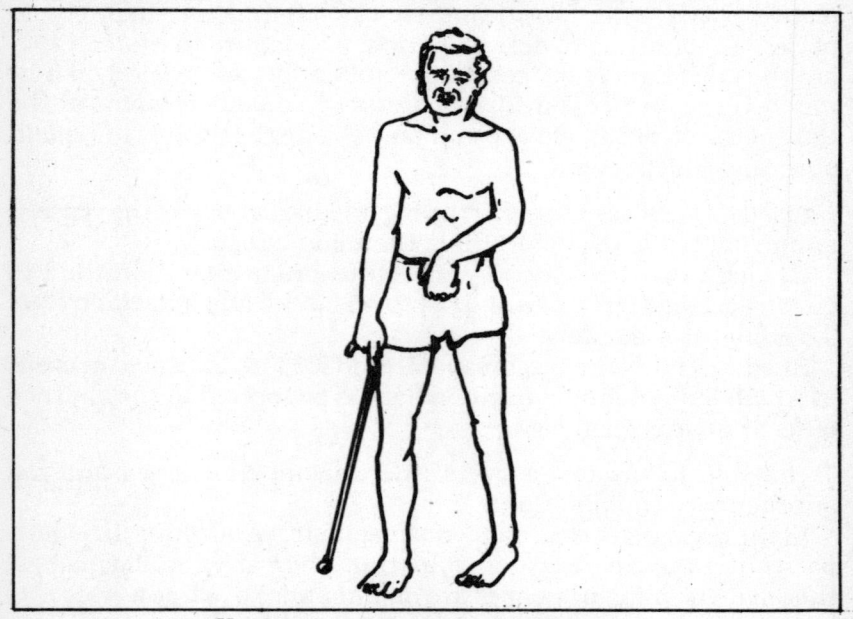

Hemiplegic patient towards rehabilitation

As regards the second aspect of treatment, namely, the rehabilitation, most major stroke survivors will have some permanent disability. The scope of improvement becomes less after about 6 weeks, and hardly any further recovery can be expected after 6 months.

In stroke rehabilitation, a start has to be made as soon as the patient recovers consciousness. Much lost function can be recovered and the same must be explained to the patient. The patient should be gotten into a chair on day one, practice balancing on day two, and stand on his feet fully supported by nurses or physiotherapists on day three. From then on, active exercises must begin with walking, balancing and limb and trunk movements.

Delirium

It is an acute response of the brain to many different kinds of bodily ailments. It may either occur in those who were previously normal in mind or, more commonly, in those who already had some mental impairment.

A patient with delirium is restless and uneasy, but his condition fluctuates. At times he may seem quite lucid, at others, perplexed, angry or frightened. He may not realize where he is, what time it is, or who are the people around him. He fails to recognize his friends and relations. He perception is distorted. His speech may be rambling and incoherent. He may shout noisily and is difficult to be confined to bed.

Cause(s). They are diverse.

Conditions Causing Delirium in the Elderly

1. Infections such as pneumonia, meningitis, encephalitis.
2. Trauma, particularly closed-head trauma resulting in subdural hematoma (blood collection beneath the dura covering of the brain), concussion.
3. Exogenous toxins, such as alcohol, carbon-monoxide, heavy meals.
4. Many drugs used for different diseases, which ordinarily do not cause such symptoms in younger people.
5. Hypoxia (lack of oxygen), hypercarbia (excess of CO_2), electrolyte disturbances, acid-base disturbance.
6. Thyroid dysfunction, uraemia, hepatic failure, congestive heart failure, hyperglycaemia, hypoglycaemia.

Treatment. The patient is often seriously ill and the best way to control delirium is to give proper treatment for the disease which provoked it. It is important also to give sufficient fluid to prevent dehydration.

Some sedation is likely to be needed to prevent the restless patient from becoming exhausted. The most useful drugs are the phenothiazine group of tranquillizers. These include chlorpromazine (Largactil) and related drugs like trifluoparazine (Stelazine). The first dose may have to be injected, but oral treatment should be used as soon as possible. These drugs make the patient drowsy and may cause postural hypotension with a risk of a fall if the patient gets out of bed. Other side-effects include a dry mouth, blurred vision, constipation and retention of urine. The older patient, with perhaps incipient glaucoma, an enlarged prostate and a tendency to faecal impaction, is vulnerable to these complications. The dose of the drugs should be kept as low as possible.

An alternative tranquillizer which calms the patient but is less likely to send him off to sleep is haloperidol (Serenace), by mouth or injection, but the risk of symptoms of parkinsonism is greater than with phenothazines.

Some patients in delirium recover their mental equilibrium within a day or two or even a few hours. Others, especially those with severe physical illness, may die. Others again, may pass into a state of permanent dementia. Any pre-existing mental impairment is likely to be made worse.

Dementia

This is characterized by permanent mental impairment. It may be mild, moderate or severe. It is always due to damage to the structure of the brain cells and their loss.

Cause(s). Two main types of dementia are described: (1) primary, also called senile dementia, and (2) secondary, after multiple cerebral infarcts, also called arteriosclerotic dementia.

The onset of senile dementia is gradual. The old person may lose his former interest in life and give up his initiative. The outstanding feature, however, is his failure of memory. Initially he forgets what has happened recently; later his memory for distant events may also be lost. Forgetfulness may proceed to a point where the patient fails to recognize people he knows well. Ultimately, he may forget his name.

In contrast to the steady decline of many patients with primary dementia, the downhill course of the patient with vascular dementia is marked by a series of incidents. Each one represents a further small cerebral infarction or little stroke and is followed by a partial recovery. Brain size and weight is diminished in dementia patients.

Treatment. A complete evaluation is needed to be done early to find out all readily treatable forms of dementia. Delay in diagnosing

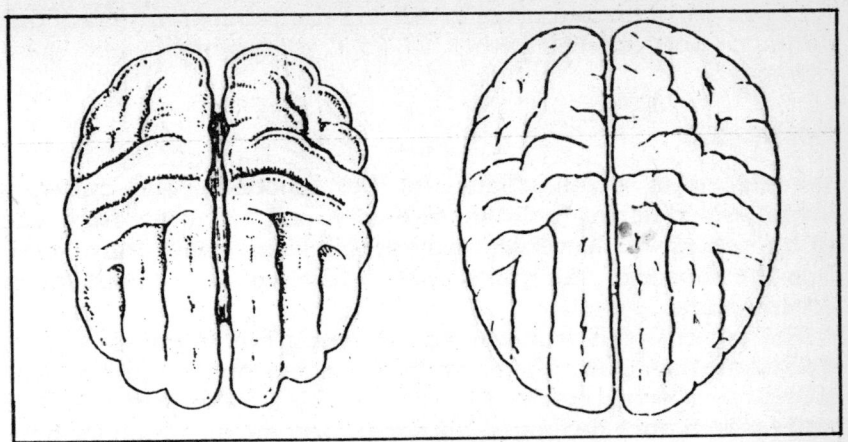

Brain: Normal and dementia patient

dementia with a reversible cause, such as hypothyroidism, may result in worsening of the condition.

A complete history including that of taking any drugs is recorded. A physical examination is done. Routine laboratory tests are done including thyroid functions, renal and liver functions, EEG and CT scanning of the brain is essential and also a lumber puncture, if indicated.

There are no drugs which have a direct ameliorative effect on the dementing process. They can only be used to treat the complications and to deal with any concurrent physical illness. If the patient is restless, one of the tranquillizers may help and if he is depressed, an antidepressant, preferably at night.

Vasodilator drugs are often prescribed in an effort to improve the cerebral circulation, for example, isoxsuprine (Duvadilan), cyclandelate (Cyclospasmol), xanthine nicotinate (Complamex), and naftidrofuryl (Praxilene). There are also drugs which are claimed to improve the metabolism of the brain cells. These include Hydergine which contains extracts of ergot and meclofenoxate (Lucidril). All these drugs may lead to minor improvements in mentally impaired patients, but none alters the clinical picutre decisively.

If night sedation is needed, chlormethizole (Heminervin) and chloral (Noctec) are safer. Diazepam is safe but addictive. Barbiturates should not be given as these may increase restlessness and confusion.

Drugs are of limited value in helping the patient with brain cell damage. Success lies rather in good management and good nursing.

Depression

Depression is a disturbance of the emotions, the patient's symptoms differing only in intensity and duration from the unhappiness which everyone experiences from misfortune or grief. It is the source of much misery and may even lead to suicide in severe cases.

The patient feels worse in the morning but improves a little during the day. Quite often sadness is not obvious, but the patient is anxious, worried or irritable. He is unable to take decisions, and tasks which once he took in his stride, become too much for him. More often, however, his misery is accompanied by agitation. He may even become confused.

Criteria for labelling an Episode as Depressive in an Elderly

A sad or depressive mood of over, at least, 2 weeks, with any four of the following to a significant degree:

(1) Poor appetite or some weight loss.
(2) Insomnia.
(3) Loss of energy.
(4) Loss of interest or pleasure in usual activities or decrease in sexual drive.
(5) Diminished ability to think or concentrate.
(6) Feeling of inappropriate guilt.

Sometimes, it may be difficult to distinguish between an episode of depression or the presence of dementia in an elderly. The following criteria may help.

Cause(s). Depression has no single cause. The illness probably results from an interaction between the circumstances of the patient's life, his physical condition and his inherited constitution. In a few cases, drugs contribute to depression; reserpine and methyldopa used for the treatment of hypertension, and phenobarbitone, are well-known examples.

Treatment. In old age, a great deal of depression results from physical illness. In addition to the treatment for his physical disabilities, the patient needs to feel that somebody understands him as a person and can sympathize with his sense of hopelessness. The drugs available for the treatment of depression fall into three groups: (1) the tricyclic compounds, (2) the monoamine oxidase inhibitors (MAOI) and (3) lethium.

Differentiation between Depression and Dementia		
Symptom	Depression	Dementia
Onset	Rapid, exact onset can often be dated	Insidious and ill-defined
Behaviour	Stable; depression, apathy and with-drawal common	Labile; fluctuates between normal and withdrawn and apathetic
Mental competence	Usually unaffected, however, may appear demented at times; complains of memory problems.	Consistently impaired, tries to hide cognitive impairment.
Somatic	Anxiety, insomnia, eating disturbances, minor physical complaints	Occasional sleep disturbances.
Self-image	Poor	Normal
Duration	Usually self-limited; reversible with therapy.	Chronic; slowly progressive

The tricyclic group includes imipremine (Tofranil), and amiptryptiline (Triptyzal). Imipramine is mildly stimulating and is preferred for the retarded patient. Amitryptiline is mildly sedative and is better for the patient with anxiety and agitation. A slow-release preparation, Entizol is available. Amitryptiline may make the patient drowsy and at times confused. It is best taken at night. The most serious side-effect of the tricyclic antidepressants is postural hypotension causing dizziness and falls. The other side-effects resemble those of atropine and include a dry mouth, constipation, difficulty in visual accomodation, retention of urine, tremor and confusion. These drugs may have to be avoided in patients with glaucoma or prostate disease. In spite of the side-effects, the tricyclic drugs are very useful. Depressed patients often show improvement within a week, but it is necessary to persevere for a month before deciding that the drug does not work. One patient in five fails to respond to tricyclics. Once treatment is established, it is normally continued for at least six months.

Monoamine oxidase inhibitor (MAOI) drugs relieve depression in some patients, particularly those who are neurotic or irritable and troubled by many physical symptoms. They are less likely than the tricyclics to help the patient with classical endogenous depression. These are seldom given until after an unsuccessful trial of a tricyclic compound because there are many problems associated with their use. There is a small risk of jaundice. They interact with certain foods containing the substance tryamine which may provoke a dangerous rise in blood pressure. Foods which the patient must avoid include cheese, yogurt, broad beans, pickled herrings and beer. MAOI substances also potentiate the affect of other drugs, including alcohol, morphine, pethidine and adrenaline.

Lithium as lithium carbonate (Camolit, or the sustained-released preparation, Priadel), was originally used for the treatment of mania. Later it was found to help people with depression, especially those prone to recurrent attacks. Over-dosage causes tremor, confusion, vomiting and diarrhoea.

Depressed patients whose agitation remains unrelieved in spite of the above drugs, need a sleeping drug, as, for example, diazepam.

Neurosis

Some older people, perhaps predisposed by heredity, develop neuroses with symptom of marked anxiety. Roughly about 10 per cent of old people suffer from neurosis, marked by anxiety. About half develop symptoms in old age, the others bring their neuroses with them from earlier life. Women are more often affected than men.

The patient may complain of anxiety and worry. He may have difficulty getting to sleep and wake exhausted in the morning. He may lose appetite and weight.

Cause(s). Hereditary predisposition and environmental factors make some people susceptible to the disease.

Treatment. Anxiety can often be relieved if it is freely expressed. A careful history and physical examination by the doctor followed by explanation and reassurance is itself therapeutic.

Drug treatment relies principally on tranquillizers. Diazepam is one of the best. Tranquillizers alleviate the patient's anxieties.

Hypochondriasis

The predominant disturbance in the patient is an unrealistic interpretation of physical signs or sensations as abnormal, leading to a preoccupation with having a serious disease. Sometimes, the condition needs to be differentiated from depression.

Clinical Clues for differentiating Hypochondriasis from Depression	
Hypochondriasis	*Depression*
Patients do not appear to be suffering despite the frequent report of physical symptoms.	Patients suffer from both their physical and psychiatric symptoms.
Anger is directed towards others.	Anger is more likely to be directed towards self.
Patients are very sensitive to the side-effects of medications.	Patients tolerate the side-effects of medications as well as other elderly patients.
A history of physical problems in mid-life is common.	Mid-life physical complaints are less common.
Social participation is hampered but not dysfunctional.	Decreased social participation is prominent and frequently dysfunctional.

Cause(s). Genetic predisposition and environmental factors, particularly stresses of the old age, are said to work as causes.

Treatment. Hypochondriasis is more chronic than most psychiatric disorders encountered in older patients, but it does not prove to be as disabling over time as other disorders.

The patient-doctor relationship is of great value to the patient. Its consistency is of great comfort to the patient because he recognizes that, to a degree, he can depend on his physician to help him.

Paranoid Disorders

Older persons often have the reputation of being morose, rigid and suspicious of anything new or unusual.

Cause(s). Paranoid symptoms in older persons may arise from several causes. With advancing age, sense organs such as of hearing and seeing, diminish in their function so that the person has difficulty in scanning his environment adequately. Memory and brain function also slow down. As a result, they react to their environments in two different ways. Firstly, they may decrease the range of their social environment to their neighbourhood, their house, or even one room in the house. Secondly, they fill the gaps in perception with fantasy. Fantasies enable them to explain situations and events that are not easily understood. As this fantasy material is integrated, it may lead to a frankly delusional orientation to the social environment.

Treatment. Developing a proper patient-physician relationship is essential. Removal, so far as possible, of the underlying causes is the next step.

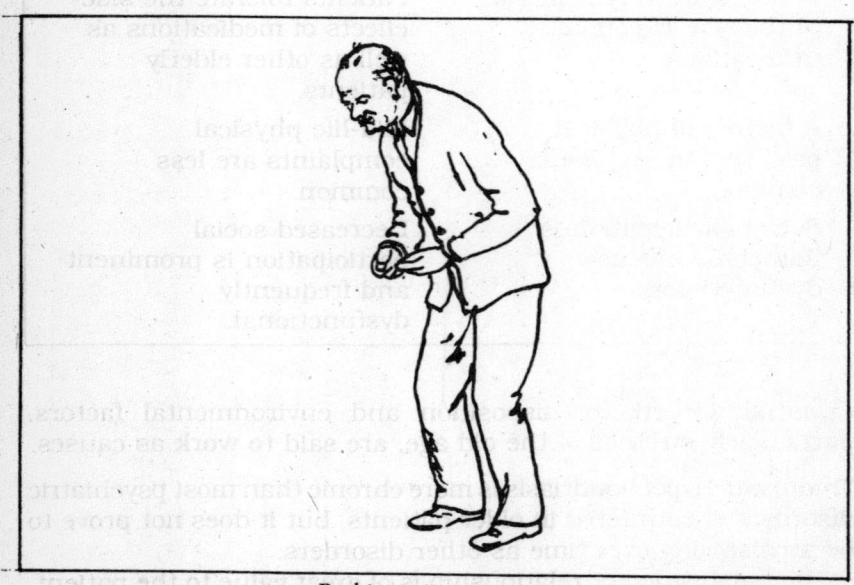

Parkinsonian posture

Parkinsonism

It is characterized by tremor and rigidity of the whole body, easily seen in the gait and constant 'pill-rolling' movements in the fingers.

Cause(s). The major biochemical abnormality in patients with parkinsonism is a loss or inhibition of activity of the neurotransmitter dopamine in the corpus stratum of the brain, resulting in an abnormal balance between dopamine and acetylcholine.

Although a variety of disorders and conditions that affect the central nervous system can result in this syndrome, idiopathic parkinsonism is responsible for the majority of the cases.

Forms of Parkinsonism
Primary cause not known (idiopathic) Parkinson's disease

Secondary (symptomatic)
  Infectious: post-viral encephalitis
  Arteriosclerotic
  Drug-induced
  Toxins
  Metabolic
  Miscellaneous: tumours, head trauma, degenerative, autonomic degeneration

The commonest cause of parkinsonism is Parkinson's disease (paralysis agitans). The next common cause is the drugs given for sedation, particularly haloperidol and the phenothiazines. Cerebrovascular disease as a cause of parkinsonism is much less common than is supposed, and most patients in whom this diagnosis is made, have had bilateral deep cerebral hemisphere infarctions, or longstanding hypertensive cerebrovascular disease.

Treatment. Tremor and rigidity are relieved by the older medicines with an atropine-like action such as orphenadrine (Disipal) and these are particularly valuable when parkinsonism is drug-induced. But side-effects are commoner with these drugs and are troublesome for the older patients.

The discovery that parkinsonism is likely to be due to a deficiency of dopamine in the extra-pyramidal system of the brain, has provided better means of treatment.

Levodopa is an effective durg in most cases. It is necessary to build up the dose very gradually over a long period. It is now given in combination with another substance, called an inhibitor, which inactivates levodopa in every part of the body except the brain, where its action is needed and so lessens the side-effects like nausea etc.

Amantadine is another useful drug. Its mechanism of action is not completely understood, yet it is felt to increase release of dopamine from the brain. Doses of 100 mg twice or thrice daily usually result in clinical improvement within 48 to 72 hours. Although it usually is reserved for early-stage Parkinson's disease, it is also a useful adjunctive medication when the usual dose of levodopa is no longer sufficiently effective or where levodopa dosage has to be reduced because of side-effects. Side-effects include confusion, oedema.

Tricyclic compounds can be useful agents in early parkinsonism. A tablet of 10 mg of imipramine or 25 mg amitriptyline three or four times a day, is the usual dose required. They are, however, poorly tolerated by many elderly, making their use less desirable.

Bromocriptine is the most recent drug used in parkinsonism . A starting dose of 1.25 mg twice a day with meals is suggested. Side-effects may include nausea, headache, confusion, dizziness, hypotension, fatigue, vomiting, constipation and drowsiness.

Patients with parkinsonism are subject to severe constipation and episodes of faecal impaction are common.

Physical therapy and psychological counselling helps. All patients are advised to establish a daily programme of exercise. Physiotheraphy is directed toward the maintenance of joint mobility, correction and prevention of postural abnormalities of limbs and trunks and maintenance of normal gait. Passive stretching of the limbs, muscle massage and gait-training are useful adjuncts in therapy.

Insomnia

There may be difficulty in initiating sleep, difficulty in maintaining sleep, altered quality of sleep and combinations of all the above.

Cause(s). Insomnia may occur in anticipation of, or in consequence of an emotionally significant event. It is by definition transient.

A special form of insomnia precipitated by loss by death of loved ones, is commonly seen in the elderly. This takes its time to go.

Pain, cough, dyspnoea, pruritis (skin irritation), and fever may cause insomnia.

It is important to consider the diagnostic possibility of depression, since the elderly commonly "mask" the symptoms of depression with physical conditions, including sleep disturbances.

The following points may be kept in mind in elder insomniacs:

(1) The total sleep time needed by elderly is less than that they had in youth.

(2) There is a tendency in the elderly to go to bed early and to wake up early.

(3) The elderly more often take mid-day nap.

Treatment. It is a matter of clinical judgment whether to use hypnotic drugs to manage situational insomnia in elderly patients. Hypnotics provide symptomatic relief at night, but can also lead to impairment of alertness, memory, judgment and coordination the next day or during the night if the patient happens to awake.

The preferred hypnotics are the new, short-acting benzo-diazepines. They should be given in small trial doses and then raised to an effective and well-tolerated level.

Drugs with long half-life or those that produce rapid tolerance and dependency such as alcohol in any form, barbiturates, metha qualone, should be avoided. The total period of giving drugs should not exceed a few weeks.

19 Urinary Disorders

It is the older patient who suffers either from retention of urine or incontinence of urine. Retention is commonly due to enlarged prostate in the males and can be cured surgically. Incontinence of flow of urine occurs more commonly in females and is a cause of lot of embarassment and inconvenience and is difficult to manage even surgically.

Ageing diminishes the total functioning of the kidneys, but unless there is an extra strain, it is not noticed. Changes in the kidneys due to hypertension or diabetes coupled sometimes with urinary infections, throw the kidneys out of gear, and lead to kidney failure.

Kidney failure in older people is not an uncommon problem, but with increasing use of hemodialysis and transplantation, the useful life of an elderly can be prolonged for years, even decades.

Urinary Infections

Urinary infections occur frequently in women, probably because of the short female urethra which allows infection to enter the bladder more easily. Elderly men are also affected.

Urinary infections may cause no symptoms at all, or the patient may feel a little off colour and become confused. Incontinence (loss of control over passing of urine) is a common symptom and in any patient who unexpectedly becomes incontinent, a urinary infection should be suspected.

Where the bladder is severely involved, the patient may have increased frequency, scalding pain on micturition and sometimes haematuria. An acute infection of the kidney may cause fever, sometimes accompanied by rigors and there may be some pain or tenderness in the loins.

The urine may look clear to the naked eye, but more often it is turbid and has a fishy smell. Sometimes, it is blood-stained.

Cause(s). The principal factor predisposing to urinary infection, is incomplete emptying of the bladder. If the bladder does not empty itself completely during the act of micturition, then a pool of residual urine is left behind and this readily becomes infected. In women some degree of bladder prolapse is not uncommon. In men, enlargement of the prostate, urethral stricture and diverticulum (a pouch) of the bladder are important predisposing factors. In both sexes, general enfeeblement and confinement to bed prevent proper emptying of the bladder, as do almost all the common diseases of the central nervous system. The presence of stones in the kidney, ureter and bladder, predispose to infection and so do malignant growths anywhere in the urinary tract and in the adjacent organs in the pelvis.

Any patient with diabetes runs an increased risk of urinary infection. The hazard of infection after urethral catheterization in both sexes is well known.

The principal organisms in urinary infection are E. Coli, Streptococcus faecalis, proteus and Pseudomonas pyocyaneas.

A single midstream urine specimen with more than 10^5 bacteria per ml, has an 80 per cent probability of identifying infection. However, it needs to be repeated, as a midstream specimen is likely to be contaminated in older patients.

Treatment. It consists in the removal of the infection by giving an appropriate antibiotic. Cotrimoxazole (Septran) is the drug of choice. This is continued until further information is obtained from the laboratory.

Antibiotics quickly relieve symptoms, but infection is likely to return unless the basic cause is also removed.

Patients with a urinary infection do better if they have a high fluid intake upto two litres a day.

Enlarged Prostate

The prostate gland surrounds the neck of the bladder in men. It produces some of the constituents of the seminal fluid. With advancing years, it commonly becomes enlarged. As it enlarges, it obstructs the outflow from the bladder.

The earliest symptom is frequency in passing urine and this may be accompanied by dysuria or difficulty in micturition. The patient has a poor urinary stream and finds it difficult to empty the bladder completely. He has an increasing amount of residual urine, which may become infected.

Patient may develop a sudden stoppage of urine accompanied by great pain. This is called acute retention. It may be provoked by infection or by drugs.

Cause(s). It is not known.

Diagnosis is made on the basis of the history of the patient, rectal examination of the prostate so as to assess its size and also cystoscopy and ultrasonic examination.

Treatment. A few patients with acute retention will pass urine if sedated and allowed to relax in a hot bath. But for others, catheterization is necessary.

Treatment of retention of urine due to prostate enlargement is surgical, i.e., removal of the prostate. Two types of operation are performed. In retropubic prostatectomy (RP), the whole of the hypertrophied portion of the gland is enucleated from its capsule. The alternative operation is transurethral resection (TUR), which is done with an instrument called a resectoscope introduced up the uretha. TUR is preferred when the prostate is small and fibrous and if there is any suspicion of malignancy.

The ability of the elderly patients to withstand surgical procedures seems to be based not so much on age itself, but on the presence of significant diseases in other organs.

Carcinoma of the Prostate

The incidence of this disease increases as one becomes older. It may, however, for long, cause no symptoms.

When the symptoms appear because of the increasing size of the prostate, they are similar to those of benign prostate enlargement, with an added complaint of pain on passing urine, which gradually increases

Cause(s). It is not known.

Diagnosis is made only on the basis of the biopsy examination.

Treatment. It consists in surgical removal of the gland. If necessary, radiotherapy, chemotherapy and hormonal therapy are given.

Urinary Incontinence

It is the loss of voluntary control over the emptying of the urinary bladder. It can lead to other complications.

Cause(s). Any acute illness, surgical operations and chronic disability, can lead to incontinence in older people. Anything which increases the irritability of the bladder such as a urinary infection, enlargement of the prostate, or a bladder stone, may as well cause it. Some drugs may also be the culprits. An older patient with severe brain damage and mental impairment may lose all awareness of his bladder until, as in a baby, it empties automatically.

Potential Complications of Urinary Incontinence
1. Increased risk of urinary tract infections.
2. Pressure sores and ulcers.
3. Depression.
4. Social isolation.
5. Increased laundry costs.

Causes of Incontinence of Urine in the Elderly
1. Medications such as diuretics, theophylline etc.
2. Coffee, tea, alcohol.
3. Faecal impaction.
4. Brain damage.
5. Urinary tract infections.
6. Bladder outlet obstruction.
7. Pelvic floor incompetency in women.
8. Senile vaginal changes.

Stress incontinence is defined as involuntary loss of urine due to a sudden increase in intra-abdominal pressure such as occurs with laughing, coughing or sneezing.

During the stress of coughing, the proximal portion of the urethra drops below the pelvic floor. The increase in intra-abdominal pressure induced by coughing transmits to the bladder but not to the urethra. As the urethral resistance is overcome by the increased bladder pressure, leakage of urine results. It may appear before the menopause, but for many women, it becomes increasingly distressing after the age of 60. Loosening of the pelvic supporting tissue, damaged years earlier by vaginal deliveries and aggravated by years of standing, becomes more marked after oestrogen secretion decreases following menopause.

The diagnosis of the condition is self-evident. The cause of the condition needs to be investigated. Rectal examination reveals impaction of faeces, as well as enlarged prostate in men, and condition of the pelvic organs in women.

The urine is tested for sugar and for evidence of infection. This may be followed by an intravenous urogram to show the function of the kidneys and bladder and to estimate the residual urine.

Sometimes cystoscopy may be needed.

Treatment. Incontinence due to acute illness, including urinary infection, does respond to appropriate antibiotic.

When incontinence persists, a number of drugs are tried. Atropine and related durgs make the bladder less irritable. They reduce nocturnal frequency. Commonly used drugs are propantheline (Probanthine) and eniepronium bromide. All cause some drying of the mouth and a tendency to constipation. They may be harmful to patients with glaucoma.

Bladder re-training requires establishing a micturition schedule and then increasing the voiding interval by having the patient consciously delay urinating. Good nursing management is the mainstay of treatment. The patient must be encouraged to empty his bladder as often as is necessary. Incontinence pads and napkins are also used.

Any smell associated with incontinence can be dispelled by Nilodor. This comes in a bottle with a single drop dispenser. One drop on the patient's underclothes will dispel offensive odours for many hours. It can also be added to rinsing water when the clothes are washed.

Catheters passed for the temporary relief of incontinence in unconscious patients should be withdrawn as soon as possible, so that bladder rehabilitation can begin. Long-term catheterization is a last resort, but it is of undoubted value when all other measures have failed.

Renal Failure

The function of the kidney is to clean the blood of all the harmful metabolic products such as urea, creatinine and others, and to regulate the level of water and electrolytes in the body.

When due to some defects in the circulation of blood to the kidney or to a parenchymal damage, they fail to perform their function, a condition of renal failure is said to have set in. The condition is also called uraemia, because one of the main products that collects in the blood as a result of this failure, is urea. This may be an acute or a chronic process.

The patient with renal failure is usually tired and listless. He is often anaemic and frequently confused. He is likely to have lost his appetite, and nausea and vomiting are common. Muscular twitchings may be noted. The patient may bleed from the nose or from the gastrointestinal tract. Finally, the patient passes into coma and dies.

Cause(s). In an already damaged kidney, uraemia may be precipitated by exacerbation of a chronic renal infection. There may be a sudden, often precipitous, fall in the amount of urine formed.

Common Causes of Chronic Renal Failure
Chronic glomerulonephritis Diabetes mellitus Hypertension Congenital or familial disease (e.g., polycystic kidney disease) Obstructive urinary tract disease.

History of the patient, physical examination, urine testing, level of urea and creatinine in the blood, help in establishing the diagnosis.

Treatment. If renal failure develops, attention is paid to electrolyte imbalance, volume overload and infection. Haemodialysis should not be withheld because of age; reliance on conservative (non-dialytic) management of an elderly patient with acute renal failure could prove disastrous.

Dialysis should be initiated as soon as symptoms of uraemia begin to appear, i.e., fatigue, nausea, vomiting and/or neurological changes. Hemodialysis can be done either in a dialysis centre or at home. Older patients, particularly those with coincident diabetes or hypertension, tend to do better in a dialysis centre. Peritoneal dialysis is increasingly popular, particularly in the elderly patient suffering from diabetes, cardiovascular disease or difficult vascular access. Although peritoneal dialysis is approximately 15 to 25 per cent slower in its ability to clear toxic wastes from the blood, fewer side effects are noted, particularly in the elderly. Progression of diabetic retinopathy (changes in the retina of the eye) also appears to be slower with this method of dialysis.

Medical management is also undertaken side by side.

Non-dialytic Management of Chronic Renal Failure
1. Control of hypertension 2. Relief of urinary tract obstruction 3. Treatment of urinary tract infection

4. Dietary
   a. Protein restriction with glomerular filteration rate
       below 27 ml/min.
   b. Potassium restriction usually with glomerular
       filteration rate below 10 ml/min.
   c. Salt restriction usually not required until advanced
       chronic renal failure.

5. Medications
   a. Aluminum hydroxide to bind phosphate in the
       intestine.
   b. Shahl's solution to treat acidosis
   c. Vitamin D to treat this deficiency and hypocalcemia.

Replacement of lost renal function with a kidney transplant is
certainly the most dramatic and desirable way of fully reversing
the uraemic syndrome. Advanced age is not a contra-indication
to it.

20 Bone and Joint Disorders

Bones form the scaffold on which are strung or contained all other structures and organs of the body. Joints provide mobility wherever they are situated.

Bone is an active tissue, always changing. New bone is laid down, old one replaced, without ever being noticed normally by the person.

As one grows older, more bone is absorbed than laid down, especially in women, making the bone lighter, thinner and weaker and thus liable to fracture. The condition is called osteoporosis.

A well-balanced diet, active movements and physical exercise keep the bone healthy.

Joints start creaking in many people, more often in obese people, after the age of forty. There are degenerative changes in the joints (osteoarthritis) and inflammatory changes (rheumatoid arthritis). There is pain and limitation of movements.

The problem with older people is that joint disorders make the person less mobile, and when they move less, their bones become more liable to fracture. Once a fracture occurs, making the person immobile, the hazards of immobilization such as the venous thrombosis and embolization, lead on to further complications.

Bone Disorders

Bone consists of protein matrix, osteoid, in which are deposited mineral salts, derived from calcium and phosphate. The calcium and phosphate are carried to the bones in the blood stream and are deposited in the osteoid by the action of osteoblasts, bone cells which secrete an enzyme, alkaline phosphatase. In health, the blood levels of calcium, phosphate and alkaline phosphatase are kept constant within narrow limits. Throughout life, new bone is laid down by osteoblasts and old bone reabsorbed by cells called osteoclasts. In the adult, the amount of new bone laid down balances the amount that is absorbed. In old age, however, bone absorption predominates, especially in women. The bone becomes thinner and reduced in size, making the skeleton lighter, weaker and more liable to fracture.

Osteoporosis

Osteoporosis is loss of bone substance, both the osteoid and the minerals. It is often asymptomatic and frequently discovered incidentially. Even the collapse of vertebrae may occur insidiously until person with osteoporosis realizes that his stature has become shortened. The most frequent symptom is back pain, localized usually to the mid-thoracic spine or to the low back. The lumbar and thoracic vertebrae are involved to a far greater extent than the long bones or skull. The pain is mainly due to associated spasm of paravertebral muscles. The absence of back pain or its severity does not correlate with the extent of osteoprosis. Jarring of the involved area by percussion, flexion or extension of the spine may elicit or aggravate the pain. In some patients sudden severe back pain due to vertebral fractures or severe pain due to fracture of the neck of femur, following trauma may be the expressed complaint. Occcassionally compression of the nerve roots from collapsed dorsal (thoracic) vertebrae may give rise to substernal pain mimicking angina pectoris or an acute abdomen.

Cause(s). Osteoporosis is an exaggeration of normal ageing process in bone. It is more likely to occur in those who are immobile for any reason, in sufferers from rheumatoid arthritis, in those whose calcium intake has been deficient for long periods and patients taking corticosteroid drugs. Osteoporosis does not affect the whole skeleton to an equal degree. The vertebrae, especially those in the thoracic and lumber spine are more severely affected than the long bones. But the involvement of the long bones is important because of the increased risk of fracture which doubles every five years after the age of sixty.

Causes of Osteoporosis
Calcium loss
Calcium deficiency
Insufficient calcium intake
Lactase deficiency
Impaired calcium absorption
Hormonal deficiency
Decrease of oestrogens or androgen hormones

> Imbalance of sex hormones and of adrenal hormones
> Excess parathyroid hormone
> Changes in protein nutrition
> Decreased physical activity

The diagnosis of post-menopausal or senile osteoporosis is usually made when the condition is well advanced and perhaps already associated with bone pain and skeletal fractures which can be seen in the X-ray examination.

Treatment. There is no drug which will ensure that more bone is laid down than is reabsorbed. The only process known to have this effect is exercise. It is, therefore, very important to keep osteoporotic patients mobile. A severe exacerbation of back pain may compel a period of rest in bed, but it is important to keep this as short as possible.

Because many patients with osteoporosis have a negative calcium balance, they should be encouraged to drink a litre of milk a day, and to take additional calcium by mouth. Calcium can also be given as tablets or calcium gluconate. Those who object to the gritty taste of this preparation, may prefer effervescent calcium (Sandoz) which makes a pleasant orange flavoured drink.

Patients are often treated also with anabolic agents which retain more proteins in the body. These are steroid substances akin to sex hormones and they increase protein synthesis within the body. Whether, in fact, they cause the deposition of additional matrix in the bones is still uncertain. Commonly used preparations include nandrolone decanoate (Decadurabolin) intramuscularly once in three weeks, and stanazolol by mouth. Women may be treated with the female sex hormone stilboestrol.

Osteomalacia

It is the adult form of rickets of the bones in which calcium is lost. The bones become soft and they bend.

Cause(s). It results from deficiency of vitamin D, which plays a major role in promoting calcium absorption by the gut as well as calcification of osteoid in the bone. As serum calcium declines, and parathyroid hormone increases compensatorily, bone resorption takes place. This is coupled with a decline in phosphorus and an increase in calcium reabsorption in the kidney.

Failure to consume fortified milk, and a higher intake of medications that may interfere with vitamin D metabolism in the liver (diphenylhydantoin and/or phenobarbital) or utilization (diphosphonates, corticosteroids and aluminum hydroxide gels) are contributing factors.

Treatment. Administration of vitamin D corrects the defects in the bones.

Joint Disorders

Elderly persons commonly complain of joint pain from a variety of causes. Early evaluation and treatment are essential in order that further damage to the joint be prevented. In addition, failure to treat joint problems promptly may lead to the rapid loss of mobility associated with the joint pain.

Classification of Joint Disorders in the Elderly
1. Osteoarthritis
2. Rheumatoid arthritis
3. Gout
4. Miscellaneous

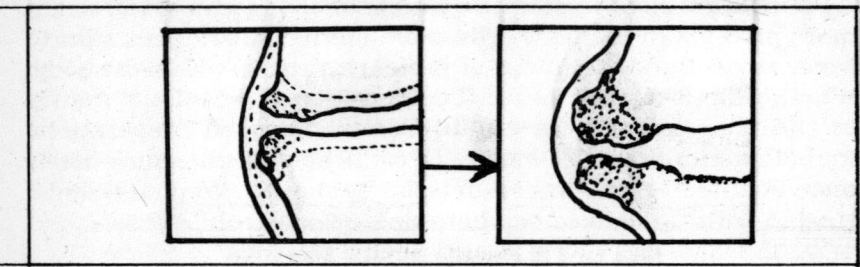

Advancing arthritic changes in knee joint

Osteoarthritis

Osteoarthritis (OA) predominantly involves the lower limb joints of the knee and the hip.

When the knee is affected, the joint between the patella and the femur is often involved as well as the one between the femur and tibia. Pain, stiffness and swelling are the usual symptoms but when the process is advanced, there may be considerable deformity also. There is usually wasting of muscles around the diseased joint, and many patients with a osteoarthritic knee, complain that the joint feels weak and is liable to give way while they are walking especially on stairs. The pain of an osteoarthritic knee is very variable. At one time, the patient may experience as acute exacerbation of symptoms and be totally disabled by acute pain and swelling. At another, apart from some weakness, disability is minimal.

When the hip is involved, however, the patient suffers almost continuous discomfort, and as stiffness and deformity increases, may become seriously disabled. Stiff hips make it difficult for him to dress and to put on shoes and stockings. To get up from a low chair becomes a painful struggle and a toilet seat of ordinary height may present difficulties. To get in and out of the bath may be impossible. Stiffness of the hips in osteoarthritis prevents the patient sitting up in bed and the deformity which it causes stops him from standing fully upright. Movement becomes restricted and the patient walks bent forward with the buttocks protruding in a characteristic way. When, as often happens, both hips and knees are involved together, the patient has to contend with a severe handicap indeed.

Osteoarthritic changes in the hand are common, particularly in the terminal finger joints where characteristic swellings called Heberden's nodes are often seen. Although striking to the eye, they cause little disability. The joint where the thumb joins the wrist is also commonly involved. The elbows and the shoulder joints are usually spared, unless the patient has injured them in earlier life or did work which exposed them to great stress.

In comparison to the hip and knee, the joints of the foot and ankle develop little evidence of painful osteoarthritis with advancing age. The ankle, especially in obese women, develops general synovial thickening, differentiated from ankle oedema by its lack of pitting.

Degenerative changes similar to those seen in osteoarthritis of the limb joints occur also in the intervertebral joints in the spinal column, but a special additional feature here is the degeneration of the intervertebral discs, the whole process together being called spondylosis.

Cervical (neck) spondylosis (stiffness) is common in elderly patients, most of whom show no neurologic abnormality as a result. Occasionally, however, osteophytes may distort the vertebral arteries and interfere with the blood supply to the hind brain. Thus, transient cerebral ischaemic attacks can occur, made worse by neck movements, particularly rotation and extention.

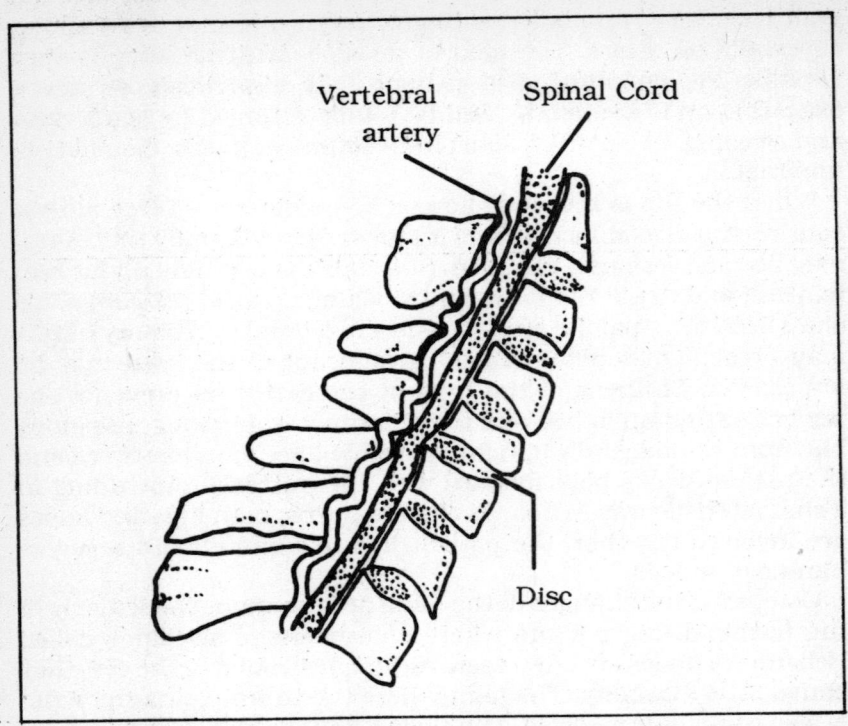

Cervical spondylosis and its effects on the spinal cord

Cause(s). It is essentially a form of degenerative joint disease and is probably present to some degree in all elderly people. As age advances, the cartilage covering the joint surface gradually loses its resilience, and this combined with trauma and wear and tear of a lifetime, leads to its destruction. Flakes of cartilage come to lie loose in the joint. They may then grow and calcify forming loose bodies which interfere with joint movement. The bone on either side of the joint becomes sclerosed or hardened, and cysts may appear in it. At the edges of the joint, bony outgrowths called osteophytes or spurs, may grow giving the bone a knobby appearance.

Osteoarthritic changes are accelerated when the patient is overweight and when a particular joint has been damaged in earlier life by injury or disease. There is, however, no disturbance in the patient's general health.

The history of the patient, involvement of usually only one joint, absence of signs and symptoms in other parts of the body, X-ray appearance of the involved joint, help in establishing the diagnosis.

Treatment. Where the patient is over-weight, it ought to be reduced.

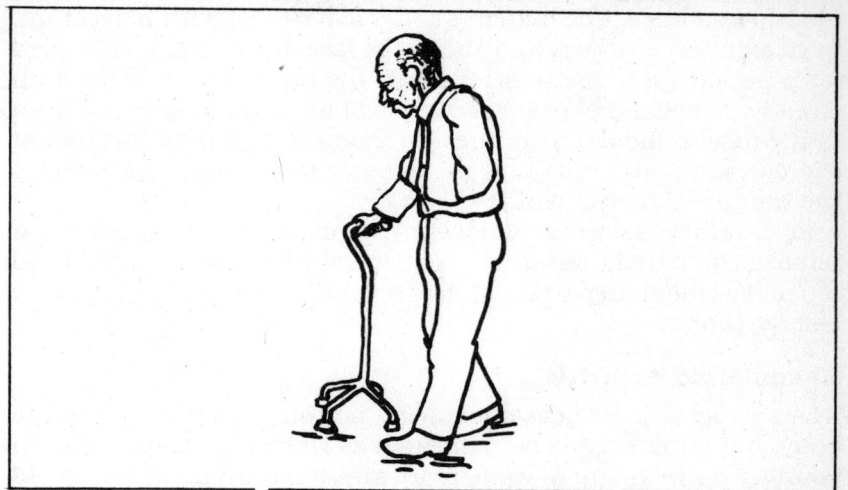

Walking with a quadruped stick

Walking aids and elbow crutches take weight off the joints and are of considerable value. Although bed rest takes all the weight off the joints, it increases stiffness and must be avoided as far as possible.

The aim of treatment in osteoarthritis is to control pain, to help the patient achieve the fullest possible function, to delay the degenerative process and to help the patient adjust to his disability. Pain can be helped by paracetamol or aspirin, as often as required, or propionic acid derivatives. All these drugs have toxic effects. They may irritate the stomach.

When there is an acute flare up of pain and swelling, aspiration of the fluid followed by injection of hydrocortisone and lignocaine directly into the diseased joint is often a comfort. Intra-articular injections must be given under the strictest aseptic precautions since there is a small but definite risk of introducing infection. A fresh disposable syringe and needle is used for each injection.

A full range of movement in any joint will produce a big dividend in terms of improved function. Therefore, great importance is attached to exercises to increase movement and strengthen muscles. Ideally the patient should exercise in a hot pool. If hydrotherapy is not available, alternative forms of heat from wax baths, short wave therapy of infra-red lamps are comforting when employed as preliminaries to more active forms of treatment. A further aim of physiotherapy is to prevent flexion contractures of the hip and knee. The patient should learn to sit with his feet up, to straighten his knees and should lie face downwards on his bed for a period each day to strengthen his hips. A patient with an already established knee deformity will need manipulation. Even in the most difficult cases, the correction of deformity, persistent exercises and attempts to walk, achieve something and keep up the morale of the patient.

In carefully selected patients, the orthopaedic surgeon can remove the patella or insert an artificial hip or knee joint. Total hip replacement, in particular, has revolutionized the lives of many elderly people.

Rheumatoid Arthritis

It is a generalized disease, involving not only many joints of the body, but other organs as well, such as the lungs, pleura, etc. In younger patients, more women are affected than men, but in old age, this sex difference is less marked.

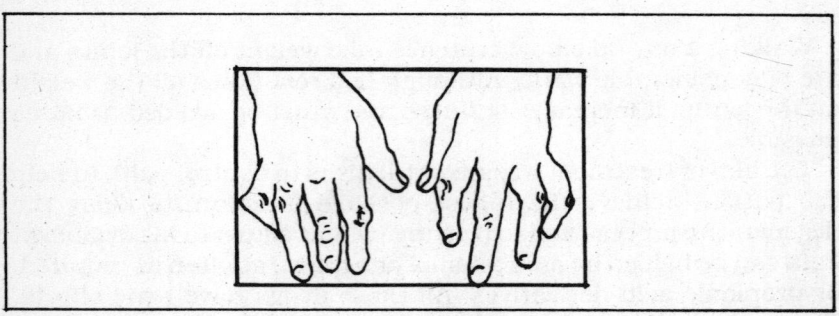

Arthritic hands

Comparisons between Patients with Rheumatoid Arthritis and Osteoarthritis.		
Criteria	Rheumatoid Arthritis	Osteoarthritis
Age at onset	Younger	Older
Morning stiffness	Prolonged, diffuse	Brief, often one site
Pain	Mostly morning	Mostly night

Number of joints	Many	Few
Joints involved	Hands, proximal interphalangeal joints Feet Knees Shoulders	Hands, distal interphalangeal joints Knees
X-ray findings of crystals	Rare	Common
Erythrocyte sedimentation rate	Often elevated	Rarely elevated
Rheumatoid factor	Often present	—

Morning stiffness of the involved joints is an important feature. The disease runs a variable course. When it is active, the patient in addition to having painful swollen joints runs a temperature, feels tired, looks ill and often anaemic. He may lose weight.

Symptoms of Rheumatoid Arthritis in the Elderly

Morning stiffness.
Joint tenderness or pain on motion.
Soft tissue swelling of one joint.
Soft tissue swelling of second joint within 3 months.
Soft tissue swelling of symmetrical joints.
Subcutaneous nodules.

Cause(s). The principal manifestation of rheumatoid arthritis (RA) is involvement of many joints. There is inflammation (in contrast to degeneration in osteoarthritis) of several joints at a time, which ultimately leads to their destruction.

The exact cause is not known.

Treatment. The aims of treatment for the older patient are the control of pain, the improvement in function and a damping down of the rheumatoid process.

The main differences from the management of OA are the use of splintage to rest acutely inflamed joints and a wider use of drugs. The management of the residual disability is the same in both.

Paracetamol, aspirin are the drugs most commonly used. Most of such pain-relieving drugs, cause irritation to the stomach and may cause dyspepsia, pain in abdomen and even bleeding. Ibuprofen (Brufen) and related drugs are often well tolerated and reasonably useful.

Two other substances are used in the treatment of rheumatoid disease. Their mode of action is unknown. One is gold in the form of sodium aurothiomalate (Myocrisin) given as a course of weekly intra-muscular injections. Overdosage may damage the skin, kidneys and bone marrow. A white cell and platelet count and a urine test for albumin are essential precautions before each injection. A patient who complains of itching or has a rash should not receive any more gold.

The other substance is penicillamine (Distamine). As with gold, its benefits may appear only after several weeks of treatment. Side-effects are common and include rashes, indigestion and loss of taste. Thrombocytopenia (diminished number of blood platelets) and albuminuria may occur; platelet counts should be done regularly. Unlike gold, the toxic side-effects of penicillamine are reversible.

The corticosteroid drugs of which prednisolone is the most generally useful, relieve pain and suppress the rheumatic process in a dramatic way. But the relief they give is relatively short-lived. They should be used only in minimum dosages. Long-term use of larger doses produces many side-effects including mooning of the face, stomach ulcers, hypertension, diabetes and cataract. They also accelerate osteoporosis, weakening the bones predisposing to fractures. For all these reasons they are used only as a last resort in the treatment of RA. They are justified only if no other treatment will help the patient. Their greatest field of usefulness is probably when they are given by intra-articular injections to relieve inflammation in a single joint. The total dose can then be kept very small.

Gout

It is a disease that primarily affects middle-aged and elderly men (90% of all cases). Onset is usually noted in the fourth and fifth decades of life, and both the incidence and prevalence increases with age. Hyperuricemia, i.e., increased levels of uric acid in the blood, often results in urate crystal deposition in the articular joints because of the relatively poor solubility of uric acid. In addition, approximately 20 per cent of those with gout, develop stone in the kidneys (nephrolithiasis) as a complication.

Cause(s). Hyperuricemia results either from an over-production or an impaired renal excretion (seen in upto 90 per cent of affected individuals) of uric acid.

The exact cause of the disease is not known.

Diagnosis is confirmed by analyzing fluid of the affected joint under a polarizing light microscope.

Treatment. Therapy of gout is aimed at treating the acute gouty arthritis with prevention of further recurrence. The level of serum uric acid is reduced by:

1.   Non-steroidal anti-inflammatory agents.
2.   Colchicine, 0.6 mg every hour until pain relief. Not more than 12 tablets in a day be ingested.
3.   Allopurinal 300-800 mg/day.

Disorders of Gait

Most elderly people in good health walk normally but slowly and with more care, scanning the ground for unevenness and other pitfalls. Some develop a trifle wayward gait with slight hesitations and deviation from the midline. Many wisely carry a cane for stability.

Anything worse than the above is evidence of a disorder of vision, of joints, of the skeletal system, or of the nervous system.

Cause(s). Normal gait depends on the integrity of many parts of the body. There must be sufficient power in the muscles of the trunk and lower limbs, normal sensation in the feet, particularly the sense of position, good coordination, good postural tone, normal righting reflexes in relation to gravity.

Common Causes of Abnormal Gait

Musculo-skeletal

Arthritis
Ankylosing spondylitis
Asymmetric limb length
Foot pathology
Shortened Achilles' tendon
Intermittent claudication

Neurological

Central nervous system disorders
Peripheral nerve disorders
Cerebellar dysfunction
Vestibular system abnormality

In peripheral neuropathy, flaccid weakness is combined with some loss of feeling. The result is a high-stepping gait due to foot-drop, a flapping or stamping movement when the foot touches the ground.

In patients having had a brain stroke, the problem is stiffness of the affected leg combined with persisting planter flexion, producing a circumduction of the leg as it is brought forward and a tendency to drag the foot with wearing out of the tip of the shoe.

Parkinsonian gait differs from any other in that the rigidity of muscles combined with their slowness of response produces difficulty in starting any walking movement. Once begun, the gait is shuffling with a forward stooping posture, causing patients to take rapid little steps to avoid falling forward.

Labyrinthine disorders originating in the inner ear in the elderly are usually vascular in origin and if acute, produce disorders of equilibrium, making the patient unable to walk at all without clinging to some solid object and progressing from one piece of furniture to another. The imbalance (ataxia) may produce a constant veering to one side or the other, and balance becomes grossly disturbed and made worse by any movement of the head. Causes in the elderly are lesions of the brain stem and cerebellum.

Observing the patient keenly when he walks, usually lets know the doctor the cause of the abnormality.

Treatment. Removal of the cause so far as possible.

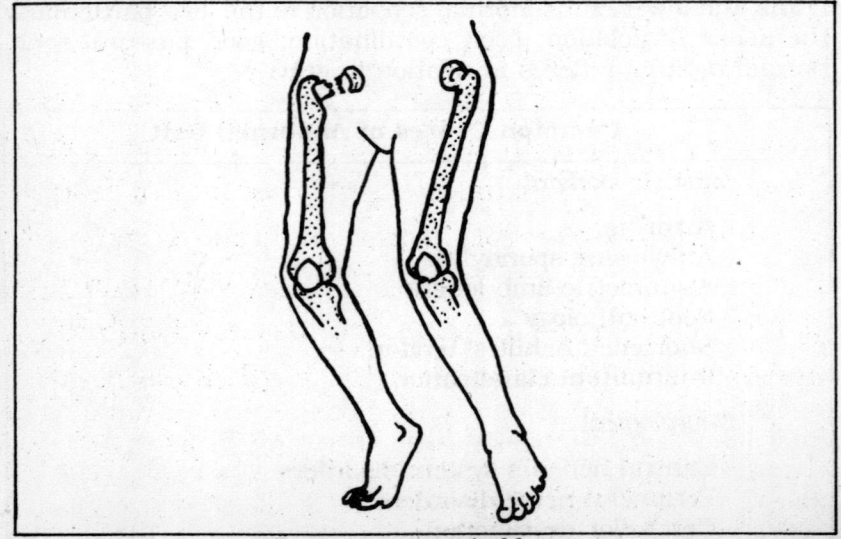

Fracture upper end of femur

Falling Down

Falls are a common problem in the older patient. They may be due to accidents, to disease or to both together. Fracture of the neck of the femur is quite common as a result of the fall.

Not only may the injuries resulting from these falls be of great severity, but in old people a fall may have the effect of precipitating a general senility due to being bed-ridden.

Cause(s). The older patient may suffer not merely from one disorder but from many: poor eye sight, defects in the nervous system, defects in the joint, general weakness. He has difficulty in saving himself should he stumble accidently, and is very liable to fall.

Causes of Falling Down
Accidental
Trips, slips and misjudging steps
Poor visibility
Over-reaching
Obstructions on floor
Medical
Drop attacks
Due to cardiovascular disorder
Postural hypotension
Arrhythmias (irregularities in heart beat)
Aortic stenosis
Due to neurologic disorders
Epilepsy
Vertigo
Parkinsonism
Hemiplegia
General weakness
Occult haemorrhage (not easily located)

Treatment. Accidental falls account for almost half of all falls in individuals over the age of 60 years. To avoid these the environment in which an old person lives, should be clear and uncluttered by small items of furniture situated in awkward positions. A second important aspect is light. Vision is an integral part of the postural control mechanism, and a dim dull light makes for a dim environment in which it is hazardous to manouver. Stairs are a major hazard. It should be clear of all obstructions. It should have a side railing and it should be adequately lighted.

It is not easy to make sure that the fall was merely accidental and not due to any of medical causes. Hence a thorough examination of the cardiovascular and nervous system is called for. If the cause is medical, then elimination of the cause is necessary in order to avoid repetitions of the fall.

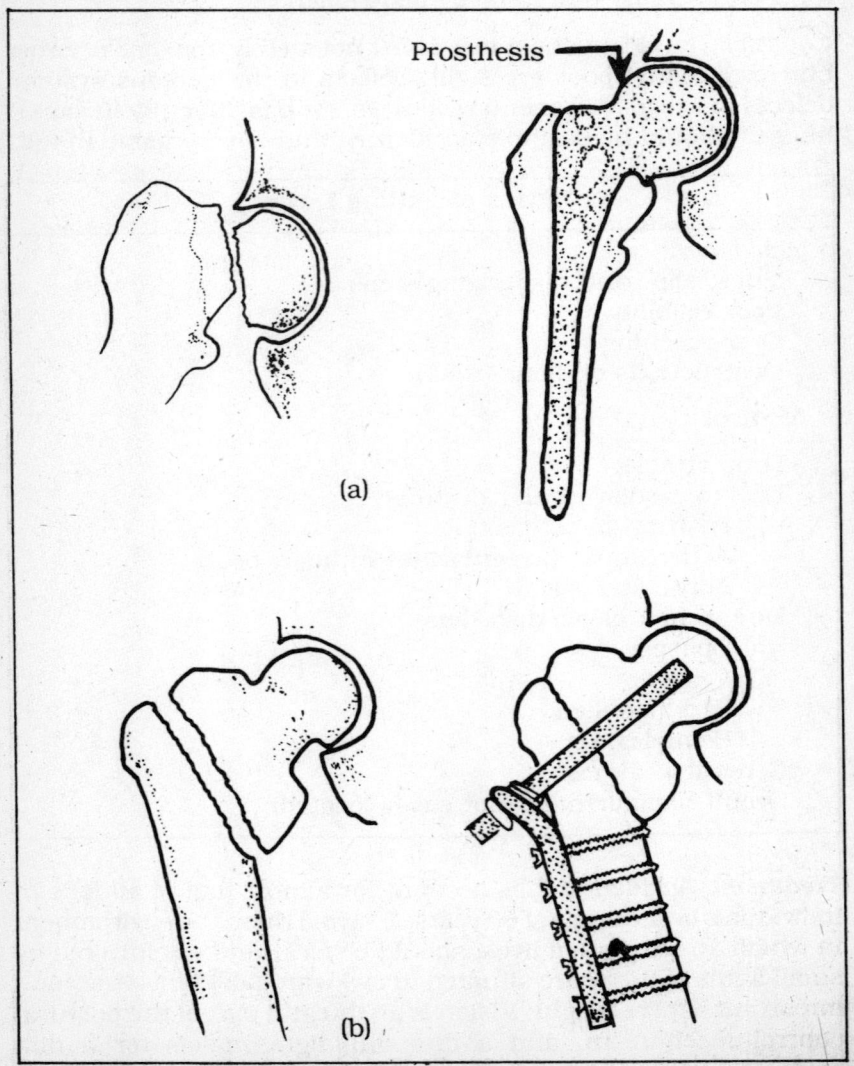

Treatment of femur neck fracture

Steps to be Taken in a Patient with Tendency to Falling

1. Review medications for their potential to cause falls.
2. Rule out illnesses predisposing to falls, e.g., orthostatic (on standing) hypotension, syncope, vertigo, Parkinson's disease, seizures and cerebrovascular disease.
3. Treat visual disturbances that predispose to falls, e.g., cataracts, presbyopia, glaucoma, and macular degeneration.
4. Advise against drug abuse, e.g., alcohol, barbiturates.
5. Periodically evaluate for environmental hazards, e.g., inadequate lighting, waxed floors, torn or frayed rugs, broken stairs, electric cords.
6. Instal safety measures, i.e., railings, nonsliding rugs, alarms, etc.
7. Provide a four-point cane or walker if an unsteady gait is noted.

21 Endocrine Disorders

Occurrence of diabetes increases with age. It is, however, not clear whether all cases having even traces of sugar in the urine or a little faulty glucose tolerance test, in older population, should be labelled as diabetes and so treated. Most physicians insist that to be labelled as diabetic, an older person should have a fasting blood glucose of 140 mg or over, per 100 ml, on more than one occasion.

Diabetes by itself does not cause many symptoms; it is the complications in different organs caused by it that lead to morbidity and mortality. Older diabetics are more often seen to be suffering from tuberculosis of the lungs, angina and heart attacks, kidney failure, brain strokes, all due to increased incidence of atherosclerosis of the arteries.

Management of diabetes in older people is easier than it is in young people, provided they are careful enough about their diet and weight. Need for insulin is less in older people than in the young.

The recognition of endocrine disorders in elderly patients requires knowledge of the changes in endocrine function that are to be expected with ageing. This applies more so to thyroid disorders, whether it is its hyper-functioning or hypo-functioning.

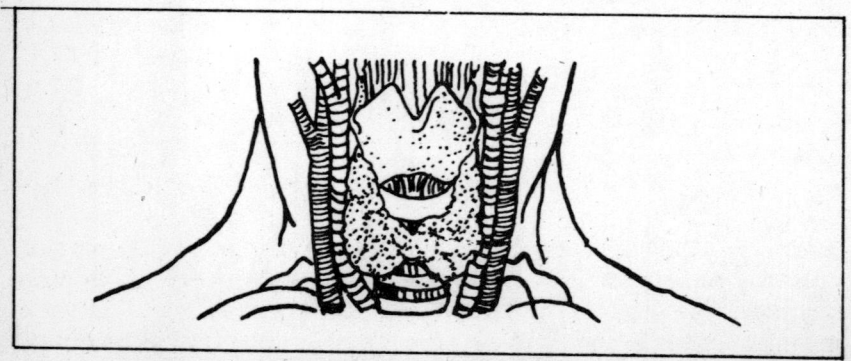

Thyroid gland on the neck

Thyroid Disease

Hyperthyroidism

Increased activity of the thyroid is called hyperthyroidism. Twenty per cent of hyperthyroid patients are over 60 years of age.

The majority present with symptoms and signs indistinguishable from those experienced by young patients with this disorder. There are, however, some differences which are important to know.

Comparison of Clinical Features of Hyperthyroidism in the Elderly and Young Patients		
Clinical Features	*% of patients having these features*	
	50 years and above	*Young*
Nervousness	55	99
Increased sweating (Hyperhydrosis)	38	91
Heat intolerance	63	89
Palpitation	63	80
Fatigue or weakness	52	88
Weight loss	75	85
Breathlessness (Dyspnoea)	66	75
Polyphagia (excessive appetite)	11	65
Diarrhoea	12	23
Anorexia	36	9
Constipation	26	4
Tachycardia (rapid heart rate)	50	100
Goitre	63	100
Thyroid bruit	27	77
Eye signs	57	71
Atrial fibrillation	39	10

Cause(s). Not known. Diagnosis is made by increase in the level of thyroid hormones in the blood.

Treatment. Definitive treatment of the elderly thyrotoxic patient with radioactive iodide carries a substantive risk of thyroid overaction, unless adjunctive antithyroid therapy is undertaken or the patient is returned to euthyroid state by the use of thioamide drugs prior to administration of the radioactive iodine.

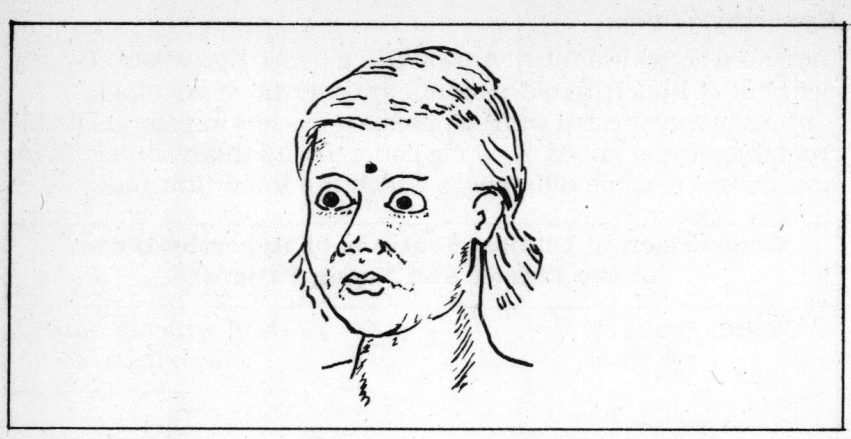

Hyperthyroid patient with exophthalmos (protruding eyes)

Hypothyroidism (Myxoedema)

Decreased activity of the thyroid gland is called hypothyroidism. Many cases of hypothroidism in the elderly escape recognition although the disease is commoner in this age group.

Signs and Symptoms of Hypothyroidism often Missed in the Elderly
Atrophic epidermis (of the skin) Hyperkeratosis (thickness of the outer surface of the skin) Coarse and thick hair Alopecia (baldness) Loss of lateral third of eye brows Grooved nails Congestive heart failure Pericardial effusion Alveolar hypoventilation Occult pulmonary infections Constipation Cold intolerance Lethargy Altered mental status

Many of the symptoms and signs of hypothyroidism (consti-pation, cold intolerance, psychomotor retardation, decreased exercise intolerance), are consistent with normal ageing and may be attributed to the latter than to thyroid hypofunction.

Cause(s). Many a time, the cause is not understood. Autoimmune atrophy or Hashimoto's thyroiditis may be detected by biopsy examination of the thyroid gland and detection of thyroid antibodies in the patient's serum.

Previous thyroid surgery or administration of radioactive iodine may be other causes.

Diagnosis can be established by estimating the level of thyroid hormones in the blood.

Treatment. Giving of thyroid extract in appropriate doses.

Diabetes Mellitus

The elderly diabetic may present with few or no clinical symptoms and signs. Frequently, the complications are the initial manifestations of the illness. They may pertain to skin, eyes, nervous system, kidneys, etc.

Several skin conditions should alert the doctor to suspect diabetes in the older patient. Generalized itching has been noted. Itching in the valua is a common complaint in elderly diabetic women, but atrophic, dry, scaly and lichenified vulva with resultant itching (pruritus) is common in older women without diabetes also. Bacterial infections producing furuncles and carbuncles should alert the clinician to suspect diabetes. Fungal skin infections like candidiasis and mucor mycosis although not more common in the older age-group, may lead to more serious consequences. Another skin lesion described is atrophic pretibial macules. When the lesions heal, they result in round or oval pigmented scars in front of the forelegs. These healed lesions are observed in elderly patients with longstanding diabetes.

Disease of the retina of the eye (retinopathy) is seen in 35 to 45 per cent of patients over 60 years of age. The probability of visual impairment, because of it, sufficient to cause difficulty in employment increases from 3 per cent in patients under 30 years at the time of diagnosis of diabetes, to 40 per cent in patients, diagnosed over age 60. Duration of diabetes is a major contributory factor. In patients with established retinopathy, control of diabetes does not appear to improve the prognosis. Hypertension may accelerate progression of retinopathy. Therefore, control of high blood pressure is an important part of the management of these patients.

The elderly diabetic may manifest a combination of nervous system disorders which include peripheral neuropathies, visceral neuropathies and cranial nerve palsies. In peripheral neuropathies, the sensory loss usually is confined to lower extremities. Pain and burning sensations in the feet with severe hyperesthesia may also occur. Absent perception of heat, cold and touch may be noted in more severe cases. Deep pain with hyperalgesia and tender muscles, is noted in advanced cases. Planter ulcers can be major cause of disability in the elderly diabetic.

Involvement of the gastrointestinal tract in visceral neuropathy is manifested by development of either oesophageal dysfunction, or diabetic enteropathy with a typical malabsorption syndrome or diarrhoea, leading to generalized weakness and debility.

Urinary bladder dysfunction may be the express sign of diabetes and may lead to rapidly developing uraemia and death. Other manifestation of autonomic neuropathy include gustatory sweating (sweating of the face and body while eating), postural hypotension and resting tachycardia. A peculiar manifestation of neuropathy is characterized by profound loss of weight, anorexia, depression and impotence. A major diagnostic problem presented by these patients is differentiation from cancer.

Diabetic renal disease increases with the duration of the disease. The clinical manifestations may include hypertension, oedema (nephrotic or cardiac in origin), uraemia, hypo-protonemia, hyper-cholesterolemia, proteinuria.

Cause(s). The possible mechanisms of impaired glucose tolerance of ageing, are impaired insulin release and/or impaired insulin action at target tissues. Other endocrinopathies associated with increased secretion of various hormones, e.g., thyrotoxicosis, hyperadrenocorticism, pheochromocytoma and acromegaly may lead to abnormal glucose tolerance and presence of glucose in the urine.

In addition, certain drugs frequently used by elderly patients decrease glucose tolerance. These include nicotinic acid and diuretic agents such as benzothiadiazines, furosemide, ethacrynic acid, L-dopa, β-blockers, tricyclic antidepressants and phenothiazines.

Diabetes detection using oral glucose tolerance tests, reveals a distinct increase in the incidence of this disorder per decade of life beginning with the age of 50. The fasting blood sugar value may

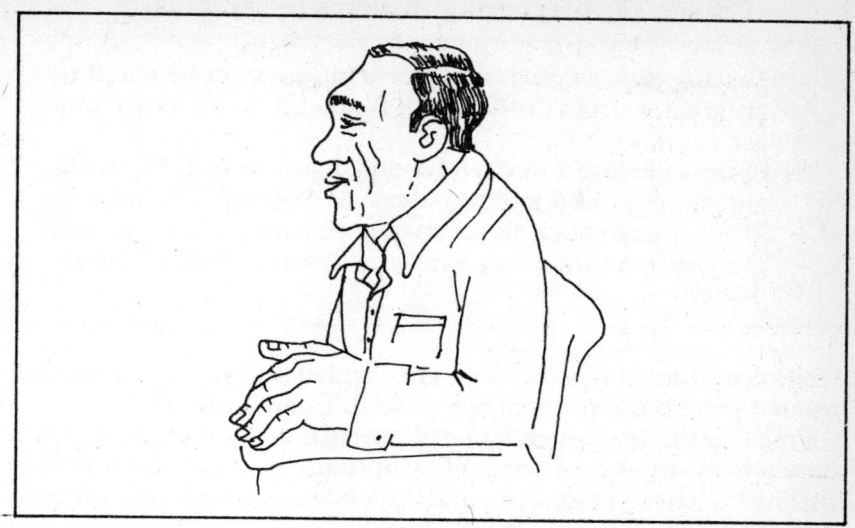

Acromegaly

remain normal, but the post-glucose level rise in a progressive and sustained manner. The result is a 2-hour sugar value that is usually as high or even higher than that attained at 1 hour.

A diagnosis of diabetes should not be made on the basis of a single glucose tolerance test, because many factors apart from diabetes affect glucose tolerance. Careful attention should be paid to the dietary habits of the patient before the performance of the test. Patient is given a minimum carbohydrate intake of 150 gm/day for each of 3 days preceding the glucose tolerance test, provided that he has consumed a normal diet prior to this period.

Inactivity is an important contributory factor in decreasing glucose tolerance. Decreased glucose tolerance is frequently noted after acute stressful illness such as myocardial infarction, cerebrovascular accident, extensive burns, trauma and surgical procedures. These events may occur in a previously undiagnosed diabetic, or the attendant stress may precipitate diabetes in a prediabetic person.

It is conceivable that the abnormal glucose tolerance may be a temporary finding. Thus either acute illness, poor nutrition, or physical activity may be predisposing factors to glucose intolerance.

Criteria for Diagnosing Diabetes in the Elderly

1. Fasting plasma glucose concentration must be equal to or greater than 140 mg/100 ml on more than one occasion, or
2. Plasma glucose 2 hours following ingestion of 1.75 gm/kg glucose (upto 75 gm) must exceed 200 mg/100 ml and at least one other glucose value during the 2 hour oral glucose tolerance test must be greater than 200 mg/100 ml.

Treatment. Diabetic patients can be divided into the following two types on the basis of their response to treatment.

Type I, or insulin-dependent diabetes (IDDM). It is characterized clinically by an abrupt onset of symptoms, lack of insulin in the blood, proneness to ketosis, and dependence on injected insulin to sustain life.

Type II or non-insulin-dependent diabetes (NIDDM). The onset of disease is usually insidious, and there may be low, normal or high levels of insulin in the blood associated with insulin resistance. Patients with NIDDM are not prone to ketosis and not dependent on insulin treatment to sustain life. They may require insulin, however, for correction of hypoglycemia if this cannot be achieved with diet or oral agents.

It is often difficult to decide when treatment is necessary for the elderly person with glucose intolerance. Frequently, the diagnosis is made only after diabetes-related complications such as infections, neuropathy and kidney disease appear, or the patient seeks medical care for a completely unrelated problem. The controversy still exists as to whether untreated individuals with mild glucose intolerance will develop diabetes-related complications.

Almost half the elderly diabetic patients can be successfully managed with diet alone. If, as is frequently the case, the patient is over-weight, caloric restriction should be encouraged. Dietary protein should be adequate in quantity and quality with minimum of 0.7 gm/kg/day of high quality protein. Sugar should be restricted. Cereals, bread, vegetables, rice should be used as sources of carbohydrate. The physical form as well as fibre content of the food may be important in determining the blood glucose response. At higher levels of fibre intake, the patient may need less insulin.

Regular exercise to the limit of comfortable tolerance may contribute to a heightened sense of well-being in the elderly.

Diet and exercise by themselves may not be sufficient for adequate control. Oral hypoglycemic agents or insulin may be necessary. Insulin is necessary in emergencies such as acidosis, infection, stroke and other stresses or during and following surgery. Its use beyond the acute stress should be made with care. Hypoglycemia may be more serious than ketosis, which is less common in the elderly diabetic.

The aim of treatment is to decrease the risk of hypoglycemia and avoid hyperglycemia. Generally, a blood glucose range between 150 mg and 250 mg/100 ml fulfils these aims. The criteria for the selection of insulin preparations in the elderly are similar to those in other age-groups.

Oral anti-diabetic tablets are given to type II patients not prone to ketosis. The combined use of oral tablets plus insulin in such patients is not generally recommended.

Hypoglycemia is an avoidable risk in the elderly diabetic. It may occur in patients taking either oral agents or insulin. Because chlorpropamide possesses a long half-life in plasma and long duration of action, cumulative effects may result in severe and prolonged hypoglycemia. However, this complication has also been reported with tolbutamide and indeed may occur with all oral agents now in use. The onset of severe or even fatal lowering of blood sugar levels in the elderly may not be heralded by the usual symptoms and signs of increased epinephrine output in the young. Many patients do not experience tachycardia, nervousness, anxiety or sweating. They become unconscious without warning. Episodes of bizarre psychotic behaviour, slurring of speech, convulsive seizures, disorientation, confusion and somnolence (sleepiness) are sometimes mistaken as signs of advanced cerebral arteriosclerosis. Nocturnal headache, nightmares, crying out during sleep, unusual sleep posture, and inability to be easily aroused, should be viewed with the utmost suspicion.

Guidelines for Managing the Elderly Diabetic

1. Blood glucose levels should be kept in a range where symptoms (i.e., polyuria, polydipsia, weight loss, vision changes) are controlled. Blood glucose levels usually should not exceed 220 mg/100 ml.
2. Avoid too 'tight' control; elderly persons are particularly

prone to complications from hypoglycemia.

3. Diet therapy should be tried alone initially in all elderly patients who do not have blood glucose levels beyond 300 mg/100 ml. Diets should be relatively low in calories, with approximately 60 to 70 per cent in the form of carbohydrate, 15 to 20 per cent protein and 20 per cent fat. Supplemental fibre may improve glucose tolerance in certain cases by evening out glucose absorption.

4. Physical activity should be encouraged as tolerated, as this helps reduce insulin requirements.

5. Before starting insulin therapy, the patient's life style, ability to administer a prescribed dose, dietary compliance (missed meals increase risk of hypoglycaemia), and ability to monitor glucose control, should be considered.
   In general, insulin should be started in low dosages; many elderly have labile levels of blood glucose, changing rapidly with acute illness, changes in diet, and activity.

6. Oral hypoglycemic agents are particularly effective when fasting blood glucose levels do not exceed 220 mg/100 ml.

7. All elderly diabetics must be carefully screened for age and diabetes-associated illnesses including hyperlipidemias, renal insufficiency and hypothyroidism.

22 Sexual and Reproductive Disorders

Social norms have traditionally interpreted the normal changes of ageing as indications that it is no longer necessary or even appropriate to engage in sexual intercourse.

Even in elderly males, beyond 65 years of age, morning erections are not uncommon. It is many of the other diseases such as diabetes, chronic kidney or liver disease and some of the drugs such as those taken for hypertension etc., that lessen sexual urge.

Many women, on the other hand, equate the beginning of post-menopausal period with 'no-sex'. This is not a fact. This period, because of absence of some of the sex hormones, has attendant changes in sex organs, that may lead to delayed onset of sexual desire, but nonetheless, the desire is there.

Older people, unless otherwise contra-indicated, may continue having sex relation with their partners, so long as the desire is there.

Male

A man's erectile capacity involves several factors such as libido, hormonal sufficiency, adequate blood supply to penis and neural regulation. Seminal emission and ejaculation are separately regulated and orgasm is chiefly cerebral. Dysfunction of any of these factors results in erectile problems.

For the male, morning erections, wet dreams and masturbation are physical signs of potency. Retarded ejaculation, lengthening of refractory periods, and slower achievement of full erection are also normal in advancing years. Insufficiency of the arterial blood supply to penis during sexual stimulation will result in erectile dysfunction. Arteriosclerosis (narrowing) and other diseases of blood vessels, especially diabetes are more common in ageing men and are to be blamed for it. Erectile dysfunction may be the first symptoms of disordered glucose metabolism in diabetics.

Impotence

Approximately 25 per cent of men at age 60, and 55 per cent at age 70, suffer from impotence.

Independent of whether organic causes are found, psychological factors can be detected in almost every impotent male. Depression, anxiety and anger can interfere with the sexual response cycle.

Cause(s). The most common organic cause of impotence is drug use. A partial list of drugs proven to cause or strongly suspected of causing, this problem is given below:

Commonly Used Drugs Associated with Development of Impotence	
Drug group	*Agent*
Psychotropic	Phenothiazines, barbiturates, benzodiazepines, phenytoin, narcotic analgesics, trycyclic antidepressants, alcohol abuse.
Anti-hypertensives	Guanethidine, reserpine, methyldopa, clonidine, β-adrenergic blockers.
Others	Atropine, benzatropine, clofibrate, spironolactone, adrenal steroids, cimetidine.

Some of the disease which older persons are more liable to suffer are often accompanied by impotence. These are as follows:

Diseases Associated with Importance in the Elderly	
System	*Disease*
Endocrine metabolic	Hypogonadism, hypo-and hyper-thyroidism, Addison's disease, pituitary adenomas, diabetes mellitus
Genital	Castration, radical prostatectomy, phimosis
Neurological	Brain lesions (temporal lobe), spinal cord lesions, pelvic nerve lesions, limbic system lesions.

| Vascular | Sickle cell anaemia |
| Mixed Chronic | Renal failure, hepatic cirrhosis, malignancies, chronic infections. |

Some of the common diseases associated with male impotence are described below:

Diabetes. Erectile failure is a common problem among diabetics. Frequency of sexual dysfunction in younger diabetic males is around 50 per cent, but it is higher in older diabetics irrespective of the duration of the disease.

Sexual dysfunction in diabetics can be attributed to one or more neurologic, vascular, psychogenic and possibly hormonal factors. Depression, anxiety, fear of complications and the daily restrictions of the disease all play a significant role.

Heart Disease. Men who have survived a heart attack or are liable to get one are often afraid of coitus and "the strain on the heart". In them, erectile failure may be due to lowering of blood pressure, systemic and penile, by drugs such as β-blockers or digitalis.

Well-treated chronic heart disease should not significantly increase sexual risk.

Chronic Renal Failure. Uraemia undoubtedly diminishes libido in both men and women. Loss of libido is often worsened by dialysis, but dramatically improves after renal transplantation.

Chronic Lung Disease. Dyspnoea is a prominent symptom during sexual intercourse. The physical requirements of coitis in terms of oxygen consumption can be considerable. Although erectile failure in men with chronic bronchitis, asthma or emphysema is common, a careful study showed that this was due less to the pulmonary disorder than to interpersonal problems created by the disease.

Prostatectomy. There is no reason that sexual activity be adversely affected by prostatectomy.

Treatment. Treatment of impotence in males depends upon the probable cause and must be individualized. If an organic cause is not visible and a psychological one is suspected, then the following four steps are recommended:
1. Permission
2. Information

3. Specific suggestions
4. Therapy

Hormonal replacement therapy, when indicated, consists of the intramuscular administration of testosterone (male sex hormone) 200 mg every 2 weeks or 300 mg every 3 weeks. Although exogenous testosterone may increase libido, no effect on sexual potency has been noted in men who already have normal levels of serum testosterone.

Female

Post-menopausal women, although still normally desirous of sexual activity, undergo changes in the labia, vagina, uterus and breasts caused by oestrogen and progesterone (female hormones) deprivation. Vaginal length and elasticity diminishes as the walls become thinner and more rigid. Lubrication may be delayed despite strong sexual stimulation. Penetration then become painful, and orgasm if achieved, may result in uterine cramps. "Coital anxiety" replaces pleasure, as the effect on the male creates a self-perpetuating cycle of disinterest. There is a fear of failure and ridicule.

Benefits and Risks of Oestrogen Therapy
Benefits
Proven
1. Control of vasomotor symptoms such as hot flushes
2. Prevention of osteoporosis
3. Treatment of atrophic vaginitis
Questionable
1. Prevention of atherosclerosis
2. Treatment of depression, anxiety, insomnia.
Risks
Proven
1. Uterine carcinoma
2. Mild water retention with occasional mild hypertension
Questionable
1. Hyper-coagulability (increased tendency of the blood to clot)
2. Obesity
3. Cardiovascular disease
4. Breast cancer

Women are often relieved to learn that the painful intercourse due to an oestrogen-deprived vaginal mucosa is eminently treatable by topical hormonal creams and lubricants.

Despite the difficulties, men and women of all ages should have the ability to enjoy sex throughout their lives.

Cancer of the Uterine Cervix

Cervix is the last part of the uterus which protrudes slightly into the vagina. Cancer of the uterine cervix is quite common in Indian women.

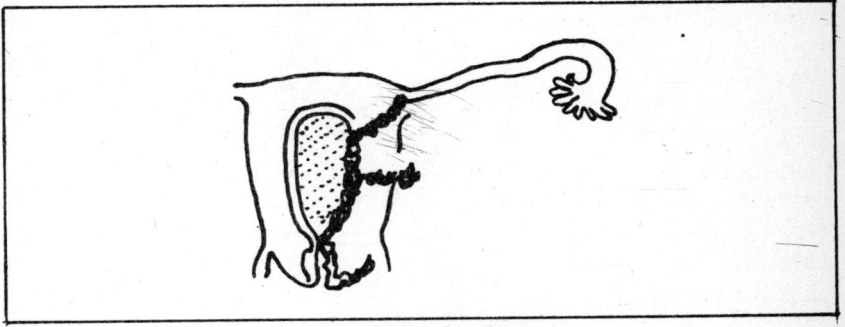

Cancer of cervix and uterus

Vaginal discharge mixed with blood occurring in women in between the menstrual period, not connected with menses, is the cardinal symptom.

Cause(s). Cervical cancer may have multiple causes. Important risk factors include poor genital hygiene, early marriage, early coitus, multiple sexual contacts and repeated child birth. It is rare in nuns, and common among prostitutes.

Another observation is that cancer cervix is more common in the lower socio-economic groups than in the higher, reflecting probably poor genital hygiene.

Physical check up of the local part gives a hint of diagnosis, which can be confirmed by pap-smear test and by biopsy examination of the local part.

Treatment. It depends on the stage of the disease at the time of presentation to the doctor.

If the cancer has involved only the surface of the cervix, **surgical** removal of the cervix and the uterus provides complete cure. If the cancer has infilterated the wall of the cervix, either surgery or radiation is done. If the cancer has spread beyond the cervix into the surrounding tissue or organs, surgery has no role. Radiation therapy is given when the cancer has spread from the local site. It is given both externally as well as internally by implantation of the radium needles into the cancerous tissue.

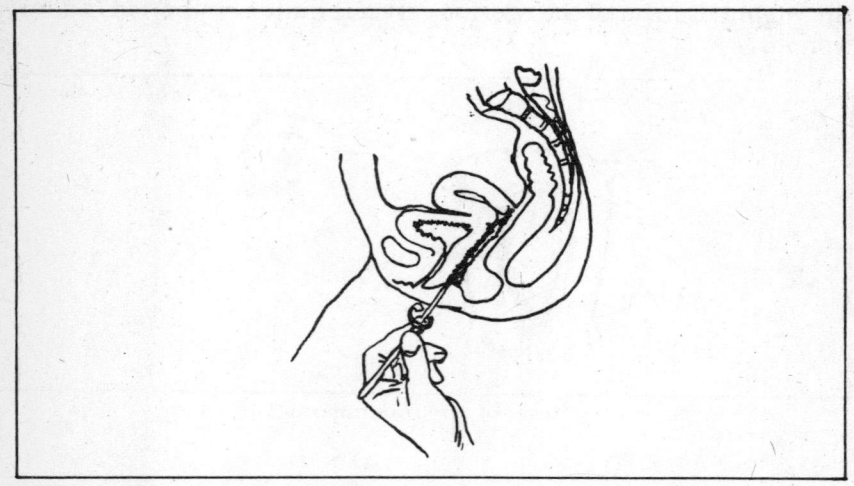

Taking a cervical smear (Pap test)

Chemotherapy has not proved very effective.

Detected and removed measure, all women going to their gynaecologist, should have their pap-smear test done.

Cancer of the Uterus

It is a common cancer of women in India. Bleeding from the vagina at times other than the menstruation is the commonest symptom.

Cause(s). It is not known. It occurs late in life.

Physical examination of the part provides a hint of diagnosis. Examination of the uterine cells obtained after dilatation and curettage provides a clue to the diagnosis. Biopsy examination can also be done if necessary.

Treatment. It depends upon the stage of the disease. Many a time, surgery, radiation and chemotherapy, all are used.

If the cancer is yet confined to the uterus and has not spread out, surgical removal of the uterus, the fallopian tubes and the ovaries is done. The results are good in 90 per cent of the cases.

If the cancer has spread further, extensive surgery as well as radiation are given. The results are good in only 50 per cent of the cases. Radiation is given from outside source, as well as implantation of radiation needles in the cancer mass so as to kill the cancer cells.

Progesterone, a female hormone, is helpful in reducing the size of the cancer in about 30 per cent of the cases. This is given in advanced cases of cancer, alongwith all the other treatments. Anti-cancer drugs are also given in cases where there is suspicion that all the cancer has not been removed.

Cancer of the Breast

Cancer of the breast occurs in women in India, usually past the age of 40 years. Its incidence is reported to be 20 per 1,00,000 women.

It appears as a lump or nodule in the breast. As this grows, it gets attached to the skin of the breast. Lymph nodes may appear in the axilla on the side of the disease.

Cause(s). It is not known. The major known determinants of risk for breast cancer are delayed age at first pregnancy, family history of breast cancer, giving of oestrogen, fibrocystic breast disease (multiple nodules form in the breast) and exposure to the ionizing radiation.

Diagnosis is established by the physical examination and biopsy examination of the nodule.

Treatment. If the cancer is detected early, surgery may bring about a cure. The whole of the breast is removed including the underlying glands.

If the surgeon is not sure that he has removed the whole cancer mass, then he may decide that the patient should have radiation treatment in order to kill any remaining cancer cells. It is given 4 to 5 times a week for 4 to 6 weeks.

In order to do away with exigency of recurrence, chemotherapy is given, besides the surgery and radiation.

It is long known that removal of the ovaries lessens the size of the breast cancer. The same result can be obtained if the adrenal glands are removed.

Nowadays, instead of doing the operation of removing the ovaries (oophorectomy), anti-hormone drugs like Timoxifen, are given in selected patients who are known to respond to such a treatment.

If the breast cancer recurs after any or all modes of treatment, the chances of cure, are not bright. However, even such a patient can live for many years.

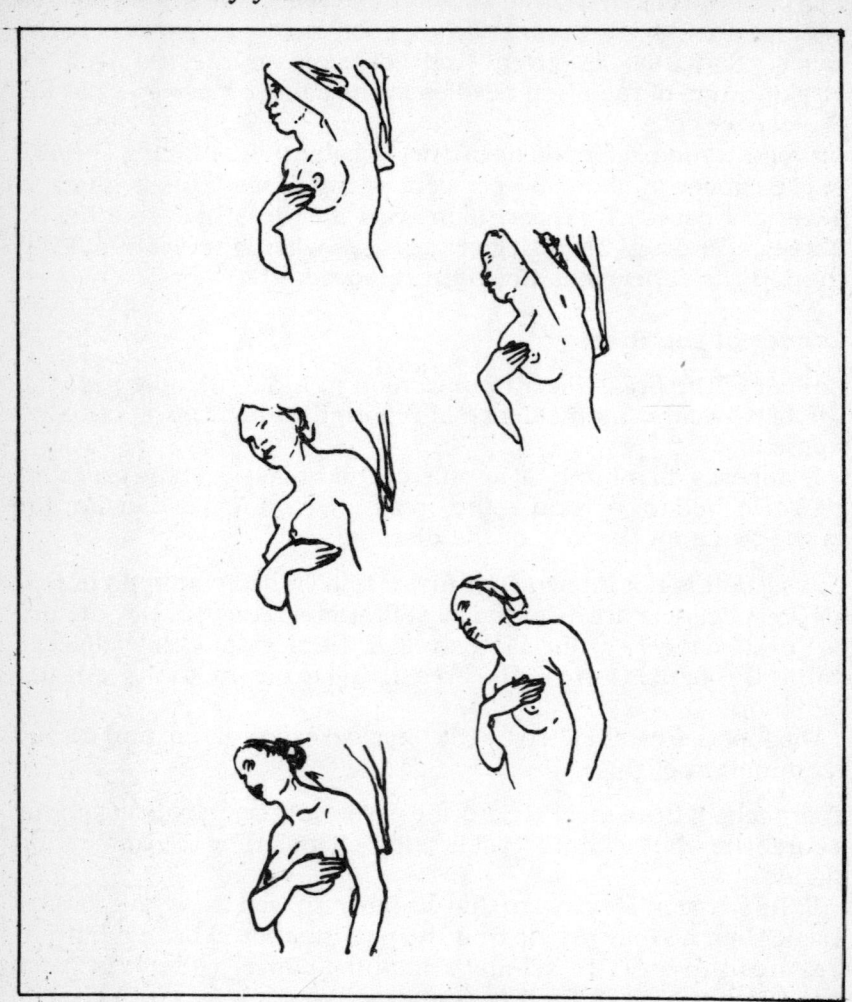

Self examination of breast

23 Skin Disorders

Ageing brings in the maximum visible changes in the skin. Wrinkles and thinness of the skin due to loss of subcutaneous fat (present beneath the skin) are the commonest. The skin also becomes dry.

On the whole, the skin in older people is more vulnerable to damage, whether it be due to scratching, infection, pressure or application of drugs.

Older people usually become careless about the skin and so run the risk of many skin disorders. The skin is not only meant for its looks; it is also protective to the body in many ways and should be looked after well.

Pruritis (Irritation)

It is one of the commonest skin complaints in the elderly. It occurs commonly along the anterior aspect of the tibia (in the foreleg). Frequent irritation and scratching may lead to redness, coarseness, and even ulcers.

Cause(s). They are many.

Common Causes of Pruritis in the Elderly
Dryness
Contact dermatitis (inflammation of the skin due to contact with an offending agent)
Atopic dermatitis
Drug reactions
Hormonal (thyrotoxicosis)
Metabolic (e.g., uraemia, hepatic failure)
Psychiatric delusions

Diagnosis of the cause needs elaborate investigations.

Treatment. It consists in less frequent bathing (water is drying to the skin), moisterizing creams, and appropriate care of any superimposed infection. Although anti-histamines, neuroleptics and other antipruritics are sometimes effective, sife-effects must always be considered.

Pressure Sores and Ulcers

They occur almost entirely in those who are ill and immobile. They may be superficial or deep.

Superficial sores are partial thickness lesions affecting only the skin itself. The underlying tissues are not involved. The sore begins as a superficial area of redness and may develop no further. If the situation is not relieved, the redness is succeeded within a day or two by blistering and this may break down to leave a painful shallow ulcer. The general condition of the patient is not affected. Pressure is the principal factor in the development of these sores. Provided pressure is relieved and they are kept clean, superficial ulcers heal readily, with or without a dressing. If the patient is incontinent, a dressing inevitably becomes soaked with urine and may do more harm.

Deep sores are far more serious. They affect full thickness of the skin and the underlying tissues. The damage begins deeply and works its way to the surface. They are caused by unrelieved pressure on the skin and underlying soft tissue against the bony prominences of the body. They occur most commonly on the back over the sacrum, on the buttocks, over the ischia, on the hips, over the trochanters, and on the heels. An additional factor is the shearing strain which occurs when an ill patient is nursed in a semi-recumbent position and keeps sliping down the bed. These two factors lead to thrombosis and rupture of the deeper vessels and thus to obliteration of the blood supply. The overlying tissues deprived of blood, begin to die, and the damage rapidly extends to the surface. An indurated mass is felt in the threatened area and soon the dead skin and subcutaneous tissue form a black eschar. Eventually this separates, leaving a deep infected ulcer, going down to the bone, which may itself become involved.

The patient with a deep pressure sore is always in poor general condition and his prognosis is bad, though mercifully he suffers little pain.

Cause(s). The risk is greatest in those who are unconscious, paralyzed or rendered immobile by traction and splits. Excessive sedation depresses bodily movement and predisposes to pressure sores, as does prolonged surgical anaesthesia.

Pressure sores are depressing to the patient and may contribute to his death. They are very difficult to cure.

Treatment. Prevention depends on the relief from sustained pressure and shearing strain. The latter is prevented by nursing the patient flat or well propped up and not semi-recumbent. Pressure can be relieved by nursing the susceptible patient in a way that distribut s his weight so widely that the blood supply to the skin is no. obliterated. The alternative is turning every two hours.

24 Ear Disorders

Diseases of the external, middle and inner ear and lesions of the eighth nerve and its central nervous system auditory and vestibular connections, are common in older people. The same ear problems that affect the young can also affect the old.

Deafness

Different grades of deafness are the commonest disorders in the elderly. It causes inconvenience to the patient and can even prove dangerous in some situations if he cannot hear warning signals.

The people who have to talk to a deaf person also feel inconvenienced because they have to speak loudly. Many a time, they talk briefly or even avoid a deaf person so that gradually the latter starts feeling lonely and depressed.

A deaf person needs to have more patience when he cannot hear well. The people talking to a deaf also need to have more patience, because after all, it is not his fault if one has to speak loudly and yet is not understood well.

Cause(s). It is commonly found as a process of ageing. It may as well be carried along in old age from youth.

Treatment. In all cases of deafness, it is important to help the patient as much as possible by speaking face-to-face and at the correct height, using simple phrases and exaggerated lip movements, in the hope that he will see what he cannot hear or get the meaning of what is going on from the play of facial expression.

Hearing aids seldom restore normal audition, even in the most satisfactory cases. On the other hand, in virtually all cases of hearing loss that do not yield to medical or surgical management, an appropriate hearing aid can be a significant help in a comprehensive rehabilitation plan.

Once a hearing aid has been selected and fitted, it is necessary that a patient learns to use the instrument and make it a part of his everyday life. Older patients require encouragement and must be taught to insert and remove the ear-mold, instal a fresh battery when required, regulate volume, and manipulate switches and controls. Instruction must be provided concerning the care of the instrument and recognition of malfunction.

The hearing aid user must learn how to cope with a seemingly hostile environment, filled with noise, unfamiliar sounds, and even familiar sounds that are not heard in a familiar way.

25 Eye Disorders

Gradually failing sight may be the underlying reason for gradually decreasing mobility. People who live with older relatives sometimes entirely fail to realize how bad their eyesight has become. Elderly patients in whom cataracts are developing may say that direct light in their eyes causes glare, so they sit with their backs to the windows.

Sudden onset of blindness in one eye may indicate retinal detachment, or haemorrhage. Many elderly patients have had no vision in one eye for many years and subsist on the other, which when it also loses sight, is a major disaster for them.

Blindness is common and a serious handicap, the more so, if it comes on too late in life to be accepted, and compensated for.

Cataract

It is the most common cause of visual loss in the elderly. Any opacification of the crystalline lens is technically a cataract but it is often visually insignificant in its early stages. Patients often complain of graudal, painless vision loss and may be bothered by the glare from bright lights.

Cause(s). In the vast majority of the cases, it is not known. Ageing increases the incidence of cataract.

History of the patient and examination of the eye by a specialist establishes the diagnosis.

Treatment. Modern surgical techniques have had a major impact on the treatment of this condition. The operating microscope, finer sutures and better instruments have enabled less traumatic surgery and better wound closure. Aspiration devices used with or without an ultrasonic device, can remove the lens through a smaller incision. The intraocular lens, implanted after the opaque lens is removed, has rapidly gained popularity over the past decade. It is usually superior to the thick lenses in the spectacles for correction. There is however, a slightly greater complication rate with lens implantation. Badly diseased eyes, should not have implants.

For those patients who originally had a cataract extraction without lens implantation for one reason or another, a secondary implant can be performed with relatively low risk if the spectacles prove unsatisfactory.

Glaucoma

The disease is essentially asymptomatic until an advanced stage. In this disease the pressure (inside the eye) rises so as to cause characteristic optic disc changes and visual field defects, eventually leading to blindness.

Cause(s). The prevalence of glaucoma increases with age, rising from a very low level in young adults to as high as 5 to 10 per cent in the eighth decade.

The exact cause is not known. Gradual loss of vision must make a person over 50 years to consult an eye-specialist.

Treatment. Drug treatment is usually helpful. Surgical treatment is recommended when drug treatment has failed or for a sudden onset of pain besides gradual loss of vision.

The basic principle of surgical operation is to create a drainage channel for aqueous humour from the anterior chamber to the subconjuctival space. Although pressure control is achieved in at least 80 per cent of cases, a significant number of patients can develop a cataract as a complication of surgery.

Retinal Detachment

Patients experiencing retinal detachment usually notice a shadow approaching the central field of vision from the periphery.

Cause(s). Separation of retina secondary to a tear or hole, can be seen in all age-groups, but is more common in older patients or those who have undergone a cataract extraction. Thus, it is not an uncommon occurrence in such elderly patients. The diagnosis is clearly made by the eye-specialist.

Treatment. Untreated retinal detachment almost inevitably leads to total blindness in the involved eye.

Treatment of most cases consists of a scleral buckling operation, usually performed under general anaesthesia.

26 Blood Disorders

Among the disorders of the blood, the commonest is anaemia. Others are white blood cell disorders such as leukaemias and disorders of the immune mechanisms.

Anaemia

Anaemia is one of the commonest blood disorders in the elderly. It may cause no symptom, or if severe, the patient may have breathlessness on exertion, and may feel fatigue sooner than other people of his/her age. Anaemia becomes a problem, needed to be tackled, if the patient suffers from emphysema of the lungs wherein less oxygen can be made available to the body, or if there is coronary artery narrowing wherein the anaemic blood can carry even less oxygen through the blood vessels to the heart.

Majority of the cases of anaemia are due to lack of proper nutrition, and iron deficiency is the cause. Many elderly have also the anaemia due to other chronic diseases such as of kidneys, liver, tuberculosis, cancer, rheumatoid disease or systemic lupus erythematosus.

Iron-deficiency Anaemia

The body's daily requirement of iron is about 1 mg but as only about 10 per cent of iron is the diet is absorbed even under favourable circumstances, a diet containing 10 mg or more is required to avoid deficiency.

Cause(s). In the older patient, iron deficiency is very common and there are a number of adverse factors which contribute to it. Not all old people like or can afford the richest sources of iron, e.g., liver, greens, eggs and meat. Absorption is made more difficult in old age by the common failure of the stomach to produce hydrochloric acid. Iron deficiency is common also in the malabsorption syndromes.

Iron-deficiency is greatly accentuated by blood loss. This may be acute or chronic. Acute blood loss occurs when the patient sustains a massive haemorrhage, for example, a haematemesis. Chronic blood loss results from occult intestinal bleeding in such conditions as hiatus hernia, peptic ulcer and malignant disease of the gastro-intestinal tract. Many old people take aspirin for various aches and pains. This is very liable to irritate the stomach and may lead to substantial blood loss, acute or chronic.

Iron deficiency is recognized by a characteristic blood picture in which the red cells are smaller than normal (microcytic) and contain less haemoglobin than normal (hypochromic).

Because iron deficiency is so often associated with chronic blood loss, it is important to test the stool for occult blood.

Treatment. The anaemia responds to iron. This may be given by mouth in tablets of ferrous sulphate or ferrous gluconate. If the patient is intolerant of iron by mouth, it may be given intramuscularly as iron dextran (Imferon) or iron sorbital (Jectofer).

Failure to respond to iron indicates an error of diagnosis, persistent blood loss, malabsorption or a failure to take the tablets, always a possibility in the elderly. Chronic kidney disease and hidden cancer may be the other causes of failure of treatment

Anaemia of Chronic Disease

Anaemia of chronic disease is not uncommon in the elderly.

Cause(s). A number of chronic diseases can produce an anaemia of chronic disease. The anaemia in all these conditions, however, improves with treatment of the underlying condition.

Common Causes of Anaemia of Chronic Disease

Collagen disorders
  Rheumatoid arthritis
  Polymyositis (causing pain and inflammation of the muscles)
  Lupus erythematosus
Chronic liver disease
Cancers
Chronic infections
  Tuberculosis
  Fungal diseases
Subacute bacterial endocarditis (infection of the inner lining of the heart)

Treatment. It depends upon treating the basic cause.

Leukaemias

Commonly called 'blood cancer', this is, in fact, a cancer of the bone marrow. The white blood cells produced in the bone marrow are immature and cancerous. They are also produced in number much more than the normal cells. Leukaemias are of various types depending upon the cell type involved and the course of the disease either acute or chronic. Common varieties present in older people are acute and chronic myelogenous leukaemias.

Untreated the leukaemias are progressive and fatal. Death occurs from anaemia, bleeding or repeated infections.

Acute myelogenous leukaemia (AML), also called acute non-lymphocytic leukaemia (ANLL) is the commonest variety among older people, accounting for 15 per 100,000 people after age 60.

Presenting Symptoms of Acute Myelogenous Leukaemia
Fatigue, pallor Bleeding Fever Infections Loss of appetite Enlarged spleen.

Chronic myelogenous leukaemia is also found among older people, accounting for 15 to 20 per cent of all leukaemia.

Presenting Symptoms of Chronic Myelogenous Leukaemia
Loss of appetite Fatigue Abdominal fulness Bone pain Bleeding in later stages

Cause(s). In the majority of the cases, the cause of leukaemia is not known. Several factors, however, are known to be associated with the development of leukaemia; they are: ionising radiation, cytotoxic drugs, exposure to benzene, retrovirus infection.

Diagnosis is established by the examination of the blood in which immature white blood cells are seen. Bone-marrow biopsy and its examination clinches the exact diagnosis.

Treatment. Surgery and radiation therapy are generally not indicated.

Chemotherapy or drug treatment is given with the intention to eliminate by killing the leukaemic cells in the bone marrow and the blood, and allow the formation of normal blood cells. The drugs commonly used are: adriamycin, cyclophosphamide, vincristine, methotrexate, bleomycin, prednisolone. These drugs are given in various combinations, depending upon the severity of the disease and condition of the patient.

Bone marrow transplant, where it succeeds, proves curative.

Advisory Hints

Hints to Avoid Constipation

1. There is no 'normal' number of times one should expect to have a bowel movement each day.
2. Stay active. Regular exercise increases bowel mobility.
3. Drink plenty of liquids up to four glasses per day, unless you have heart, circulatory or kidney problems. In that case, discuss fluid intake with your physician.
4. Do not neglect the 'urge' to defecate.
5. Try emptying your bowels at a preset time each day.
6. Take advantage of the normal 'gastrocolic reflex'; try emptying your bowels 10 to 20 minutes after a hot drink, breakfast or dinner.
7. Allow adequate time for bowel movements.
8. Foods containing fibres (15 to 30 gm/day) improve bowel function.
9. Try eating fewer highly processed foods such as sweets and fewer foods that are high in fat.
10. Avoid use of laxatives and/or enemas.
11. If bowel movements continue to be a problem, see your physician.

Hints to Improve Your Memory

1. Be alert and aware. Anything you wish to remember, you must first observe carefully. When you really pay attention, you will become aware of things that ordinarily might make only a vague impression. Since concentration is essential to improving memory, make sure that you are concentrating on one thing at a time and that all form of distraction are minimized.

2. Link ideas to images. All memory is based on associating new information to some thing that you already know. In improving memory, the trick is to link what you want to remember to a strong visual image.

3. Cure absent-mindedness. Forgetting to turn the gas off or misplacing a set of keys is basically a memory problem. The cure is the trick of association. A timer can help remind you when to turn the gas off, and associating important items, such as keys with specific places in the home can be helpful. For example, you might hang keys on the door knob. Thus, you always associated the door knob with your keys.

4. Be orderly. Forming good habits around the home can help to counteract memory lapses. Medications or dentures should always be kept in the same place. Making lists of things to remember is helpful, as are calendars for remembering birthdays and anniversaries.

5. Repeat three times. Studies have shown that for most people a new piece of information must be repeated at least three times before it becomes fixed in the memory bank. Some people need as many as 16 repetitions, irrespective of the age. For an even stronger impression of the memory, the idea should be repeated verbally and linked to some visual image.

6. Organize new information. New information can be remembered more easily if it is organized into categories. Either a mental or written outline can serve as a memory cue. A speech or a lesson can always be remembered more easily if it is arranged in a logical order with particular subheading. Organization can also involve words that help you remember.

7. Relax and take your time. Memory functions best when you are relaxed and can concentrate. When you are tense, tired or emotionally upset, you cannot expect optimal memory function. Older people cannot absorb too much new

information at one time and they may take more time to do so than a younger person. For them, learning just a little at a time may be helpful. If you are unable to recall relatively unimportant information, you should try to avoid anxiety. If you take your mind off it, it very likely will come to you at a later time.

Hints about Avoiding Accidents at Home

1. Illuminate all stairways and provide light switches at both top and bottom.

2. Provide night lights or bedside light switches.

3. Stairs should preferably have handrails and at proper height.

4. Carpets must be tacked down.

5. Furniture and other objects must be arranged so that they do not obstruct frequently travelled pathways.

6. Non-skid mats or strips should be used in the bath room.

7. Outdoor steps and walkways must be well lighted and in good repair.

8. Never smoke in bed or when tired.

9. When in the kitchen, do not wear flammable, clothing.

10. An emergency exit route should be planned and well understood by all household members.

11. Locks should be secure yet easy to open in times of emergency.

12. Keep emergency telephone numbers readily accessible.

13. Do not climb on ladders, tables or chairs.

14. Use step stools only according to specification and only if not alone.

15. Keep off wet floors. Shoes must be well secured and low healed.

16. Long clothing may also result in falls.

Hints to Make Your Kitchen a Safer Place

1. Place all shelves at eye level or put commonly used food on the counter. Items in the refrigerator should be stored within easy access.

2. Avoid excessive bending or reaching. Use of chairs and ladders can be dangerous. Step stools must be sturdy.

3. All chairs should have heavy backs, arm rests, and non-slip legs. The seat should be of appropriate height to allow easy ability to get on and off the chair.

4. Clean up spills promptly.

5. Use *chappals* with non-skid soles.

6. Have adequate lighting in the kitchen, especially around cooking and cutting areas.

7. Do not wear long or loose clothing in the kitchen. Clothing should be made of non-inflammable materials. Plastic aprons can be hazardous.

8. Store all appliances, utensils, and cooking accessories in secured and marked areas.

9. A fire extinguisher should be within easy reach.

10. Have emergency telephone numbers pasted near the kitchen telephone.

Old Man, Know Thy Limitations

Food

1. Do not try to bite or break hard objects with your teeth. Your teeth may break.
2. Try to eliminate deep-fried things from your food.
3. Take at least 1/2 litre of milk daily.
4. Take a little less quantity of diet than your stomach demands or your tongue relishes. Do not over-eat.
5. You should supplement your diet with a tablet of multivitamins and minerals.
6. Avoid alcohol.
7. Stop smoking, if you are a smoker.

Physical Exercise

1. Take morning walk daily.
2. Physical exercise or Yoga exercises must be done daily. If you have not done so before, start slowly and gradually.

Taking Medicines

1. Long years of taking medicines for various ailments have not made you expert in the field. Take the advice of the doctor, if you do not feel well.
2. Throw away the long-kept medicines in your cup-board or drawers.
3. Remember, youth cannot be brought back. Use of excitatory drugs, stimulants, hormones or aphrodisiacs increases the wear and tear of the body.
4. Avoid darkening your hair with any chemical solution, if it causes irritation in your scalp.
5. Avoid use of sleeping pills as far as possible.

Avoiding Accidents

1. Cross the road very carefully. Your strength and your reflexes are weak now, and they may leave you in lurch in the middle of the road.
2. Walk carefully. Scan the ground for any depressions, pits or obstructions.
3. Better avoid climbing the ladders or high stools.

Reduce Obesity

1. Obesity increases chances of getting accidents.
2. Obesity increases chances of suffering from:
    Diabetes
    Hypertension
    Arthritis
3. Obesity reduces life-span.
    So try to bring back your weight to normal or within + 10 per cent of your age.

Daily Routine

Take a short nap after lunch.

Consulting your doctor

1. If you do not feel well, see your doctor and follow his advice.
2. Get your teeth and gums checked up and properly conditioned at least once a year.
3. Get your vision tested, if you have difficulty reading.
4. Get yourself physically checked up yearly.
5. If your doctor advises, get your blood tested for haemoglobin, urine for routine examination including albumin and sugar and ECG if indicated.
6. Women above 40, should get Pap-Cervical smear test done yearly.
7. Women above 40, should learn to examine their breasts fortnightly according to instructions set out elsewhere in the book.

Planning

1.
    Plan your day.
2. Plan your week, month and year. Plan the next decade as to what you intend to achieve.
3. Try not to fritter away your time and energy in only day-to-day work.
4. Try to reduce unnecessary speech, thought and action. Learn to sit in meditation.
5. Think how you wish to be remembered after death and what you have to do now in this regard.
6. Try more to give, rather than to get.

GLOSSARY

Achilles' tendon

Tendon is a cord of tissue that connects a muscle with a bone. Achilles' tendon connects the back of the foot bone with the strong muscle at the back of the leg. Achilles in Greek mythology was a giant who could not be killed until he was hit with an arrow at the tendon named after it.

Acid-base equilibrium

Cells of the body function best at a particular pH of the blood. This level of pH, usually of 7.4, is maintained in the body with the help of kidneys, lungs, etc.

Acromegaly

The term means enlargement of the terminal parts of the body. In this condition, there may be enlargement of the nose, maxilla, mandible, hands, feet. There may also be an increase in length of the body, if the condition occurs before the growth of the body has stopped. It is a pituitary gland disorder.

Adams-Stokes attacks

Named after the two doctors Adams and Stokes who described and elucidated these attacks. Herein the rate of the heart beat is reduced drastically and less blood goes to the brain, sometimes leading to unconsciousness.

Adreno cortico steroids

Hormonal secretions of the cortex of the adrenal gland. These have been synthesized and are given as anti-inflammatory agents against various diseases, such as asthma.

Aerobic	Any process that takes place in or makes use of oxygen.
Albuminuria	Presence of albumin in the urine. It indicates abnormality in the functioning of the kidneys.
Anaerobic	Any process that does not need the use or presence of oxygen.
Antibiotics	Drugs derived from living micro organisms, such as penicillin, streptomycin, etc.
Arteriosclerosis	Hardening of the arteries, usually due to deposition of fatty material in their walls.
Ataxia	An unbalanced posture.
Atelectasis	Airlessness of a part or whole of a lung. This may be due to blocking of the bronchus from inside or pressure on the bronchus from outside.
Atherosclerosis	Deposition of fatty material, usually in the wall of the blood vessels, making them narrow.
Atrophy	Degeneration due to not being put to use.
Auricles	Upper two chambers of the heart.
Auricular fibrillation	In this condition, instead of the regular contraction of about 70 times per minute, the auricles of the heart just fibrillate, and so are unable to push the blood into the ventricles.
Biopsy	Removal and histological examination of a diseased tissue or organ.
Bronchitis	Inflammation of the bronchi, the airways in the lungs.
Bronchoscopy	Seeing directly into the bronchi through a lighted tube, called bronchoscope. Nowadays, instead of a rigid metallic tube, a flexible fibreoptic bronchoscope is used, so that its insertion into the bronchi is less uncomfortable to the patient.

Calcium-channel blockers	Drugs which block the entry of calcium into the cells from the extracellular fluid. They lower the excitability of the cells. They decrease the rate of heart beat and the demand of oxygen by the heart muscle.
Calcification	Deposition of calcium.
Cardiac output	It is the quantity of blood per minute carried out of the heart into the aorta when the left ventricle contracts.
Cartilage	Firm elastic tissue that joins one bone with the other. As one advances in age, it gets calcified.
Cataract	Opacity in the lens of the eye ball.
Catecholamines	Chemicals liberated by the adrenals and allied tissues, whose increased quantity in the blood raises the blood pressure.
Catheter	A flexible rubber or polythene tube for insertion into an internal organ or part of the body.
Cerebral hypoxia	Availability of less than normal quantity of oxygen to the brain.
Chemotherapy	Treatment with a chemical. The term usually refers to the drug treatment of cancer.
Chromatin	Material in the nucleus of a cell which carries hereditary characteristics.
Chronic corpulmonale	Chronic damage to the heart from a disease originating in the lungs.
Cirrhosis	Fibrosis of the liver, so that there are fibrous strands in places where the liver cells should be. The liver functioning is markely by deranged.
Cochlea	Part of the inner ear concerned with hearing.
Collagen disorders	Collagen is a complex material present between the cells in the body. If it is

deranged chemically, it affects all parts of the body.

Congestive heart failure Failure of function of both the ventricles of the heart, causing swelling of the body, breathlessness and bluish coloration (cyanosis) of the body.

Contrast arteriography Visualization of an artery on a television screen, after having injected into it a drug that makes the artery visible, when the blood is passing through it.

Coronary artery bypass surgery In this surgical procedure, the blocked portion/s of the coronary arteries of the heart are replaced with a vein, so that the circulation of blood to the heart muscle is restored.

Creatinine clearance It is a test to assess the functioning of the kidneys. It shows how much the kidneys can clear the blood of the creatinine present in it and throw it out in the urine.

CT scanning This is a technique by which paper-thin sections of an organ or tissue can be examined and X-rayed on a film. It is a great help in diagnosis of diseases.

Dehydration A condition in which water has been drained out of the cells of the body so that they do not function well. This usually occurs when excessive water is lost through diarrhoea or vomiting.

DNA Deoxyribonucleic acid. A constituent of the cell nucleus concerned with genetic characteristics.

Diuretic Which causes increased formation and excretion of urine.

Diverticulitis Inflammation in an abnormally produced pouch (diverticulum) in the wall of the intestine.

Electrolyte imbalance	Cells in the body function optimally when sodium, potassium, calcium, etc. (electrolytes) are present in proper quantities inside and outside them. If this balance is disturbed. they do not function normally.
Embolism	Partial or complete obstruction of a blood vessel, the obstructing mass having arrived from some distant place.
Emphysema	Over-inflation of the terminal parts of the lungs, the alveoli.
Erythrocyte sedimentation rate	Rate of sedimentation of red blood cells as observed in a tube. These cells settle down faster in many inflammatory conditions of the body.
Fistula	A long pipe-like ulcer with narrow mouth, sometimes seen at the lower end of the anus. It may be very painful.
Fungal diseases	Diseases caused by fungi or moulds, such as the thrush in children or the skin or nail infections. Some of these diseases also involve internal organs, particularly in patients having low resistance or immunity.
Furosemide	A type of diuretic which leads to a larger quantity of urine being passed. It causes more loss of sodium in the urine and so lowers blood pressure.
Glaucoma	Raised pressure in the eye ball, which can cause degeneration of the optic nerve due to increased pressure on it.
Glomerulus	Uppermost part of the nephron, the unit of kidney, which consists of a cluster of capillaries through which the blood filters in, ultimately to form urine.
Glucagon	A hormonal secretion of the pancreas whose action in a general way is opposite to that of insulin.

Heart-burn	Burning sensation in the lower part of the chest. It is usually not due to an abnormality of the heart, but is associated with inflammation of the stomach or the duodenum.
Heberden's nodes	Hard nodules usually seen on or near the finger-joints in older people suffering from rheumatoid arthritis.
Hemiplegia	Paralysis of one half of the body.
Hernia	Protrusion of an organ into an abnormal place through a broken wall, such as the inguinal hernia, umblical hernia, etc.
Hormone	A secretion of some glands of the body such as of adrenals, pituitary, etc., which is poured directly into the blood and regulates a particular function of the body.
Hyperglycaemia	A state of more than normal glucose or sugar in the blood, as occurs in diabetes.
Hypertrophy	Excessive growth due to over-stimulation
Hypoglycaemia	A state of less than normal glucose in the blood, as can happen in a diabetic patient given an excessive amount of insulin injection.
Hypoxia	A state of less than normal oxygen in the blood, and the tissues and organs.
Immune	Having resistance (immunity) against a germ. This immunity may be hereditary or acquired, active or passive.
Immune-deficiency	Deficiency of resistance (immunity) against germs. This may be hereditary or acquired.
Incontinence	Deficiency of self-restraint in passing urine or faeces.
Jaundice	Yellow coloration of the skin. This may be an indication of an abnormal functioning of the liver.

Kidney function tests	Tests performed to assess whether the kidneys are functioning normally or not. These include estimating the level of blood urea, glomerular filteration, creatinine clearance, etc.
Kyphosis	Permanent bending forward of the trunk, often seen in older people.
Left ventricular failure	Failure of the left ventricle to push out blood in the aorta, needed for nourishment of all parts of the body.
Libido	Emotional craving prompting sexual activity.
Lipidemia	Increased quantities of different types of fat in the blood, such as cholesterol, low and high density lipo-proteins.
Liver function tests	Tests performed to see whether the liver is functioning normally or not. These include the level of bilirubin in the blood, some enzymes such as SGOT, SGPT, etc.
Lung function tests	Tests performed to see whether the lungs are functioning normally or not. These include spirometry, air-flows, diffusion of gases, and estimation of oxygen and carbon dioxide in the blood.
Mammogram	A special type of X-ray investigation to detect early breast cancer.
Myocardial infarction	Death of a part of the heart muscle which has been deprived of its blood supply due to a blockage in its passage.
Occult blood in stool	Blood that is not visible as clear blood. If bleeding occurs into the intestinal tract somewhere high up in the stomach or duodenum, by the time it appears at the anus, it can, however, be detected by chemical tests.

Pancreatic duct	Channel from the pancreas that collects its secretion and pours it into the duodenum.
Paroxysmal atrial tachycardia	Sudden onset of rapid beating of the heart upto 100 to 150 times in a minute.
Polycythemia	Increased number of all types of cells in the body.
Polydipsia ia	Excessive thirst, as happens in diabetes.
Polyphagia	Excessive appetite as happens in diabetes.
Polyuria	Passing excessive quantity of urine, as happens in diabetes.
Radiation therapy	Treatment with X-rays. This treatment kills susceptible cancer cells, but also damages some of the normal exposed cells.
Raynaud's phenomenon	Blanching or cyanosis of the part of the body on immersion in cold water.
Reflex action	Sudden activity in a part of the body, as for example, narrowing of the pupil of the eye on exposure to strong light. It is a protective mechanism but gets sluggish as one ages. The impulse for action travels in the nerve pathways.
Renal dialysis	When the kidneys fail to perform their function, urea and other harmful excretory products collect in the blood and the body. If they are not removed, death ensues. Through dialysis (peritoneal or hemodialysis), these harmful substances are removed, so that the patient's life is prolonged, till kidney transplant can take place.
Respiratory insufficiency	Insufficiency in exchange of gases in the lungs so that more carbon dioxide and less oxygen than normal is present in the blood.

Rheumatoid factor	It is a protein, a type of gamma globulin in the blood, found more often in patients suffering from rheumatoid arthritis.
Right ventricular failure	Failure of the right ventricle to push out blood in the pulmonary artery for oxygenation in the lungs.
RNA	Ribonucleic acid. A constituent of the cell nucleus concerned with protein synthesis.
Subcutaneous fat	Fat beneath the skin.
Syncope	Fainting due to fall in blood pressure.
Thrombus	Partial or complete obstruction of a blood vessel, the obstructing mass being formed locally.
Thrombo-embolism	Partial or complete obstruction of a blood vessel, the obstructing mass being formed locally as well as coming as an embolus from a distant place.
Thyroid function tests	Tests performed to assess the functioning of the thyroid. These include estimating the various thyroid hormones in the blood, the uptake of radioactive iodine and scanning of the thyroid.
Tranquillizer	Drug which brings about tranquillity. These drugs are habit-forming.
Ultrasonography	Visualization of an internal part of the body on a television screen by the use of very high frequency sound waves.
Uraemia	A state of more than normal urea in the blood. this is due to failure of kidney function.
Urinalysis	Analysis of urine. Urine examination.
Varicose veins	A condition in which the veins look like a bag full of worms. It is usually seen on the back of the clves in the legs.
Ventricles	Lower two chambers of the heart.

Index